Debbie Hardy has written a down-to-earth, practical guide for those embarking on the journey through cancer and for their caregivers. She speaks as one who has been down the path and shares words of wisdom earned through hard work, tears, and love for her husband. Debbie's warm style and desire to explain difficult topics in an easy-to-understand format will serve as a road map for the difficult days ahead. The voice of experience speaks loudly yet tenderly through every page. This book will be a handy guide and valuable resource for a long time to come.

— JOANNE RUCH, MD

Stepping Through cancer

A Guide for the Journey

A MUST-READ
WHEN SOMEONE YOU
LOVE IS DIAGNOSED

Stepping Through cancer

A GUIDE
for the
JOURNEY

DEBORAH HARDY

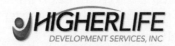

DEVELOPMENT SERVICES, INC

Oviedo, Florida

Stepping Through Cancer—A Guide for the Journey
by Deborah Hardy

Published by HigherLife Development Services, Inc.
400 Fontana Circle
Building 1 – Suite 105
Oviedo, Florida 32765
(407) 563-4806
www.ahigherlife.com

ISBN 13: 978-1-935245-38-4
ISBN 10: 1-935245-38-4

Cover Design: r2cdesign—Rachel Lopez
Cover photo by Martyn Davies; back cover photo by Brian D. Harmon.

First Edition
10 11 12 13 — 9 8 7 6 5 4 3 2 1
Printed in the United States of America

This book is dedicated to

my wonderful husband, Bryan,
who shared his journey with me
and provided the hope and opportunity
for me to write this book,

and to Mark Cerdena,
who gave us courage for our journey.

In his heart a man plans his course,
but the L<small>ORD</small> *determines his steps.*

Proverbs 16:9

TABLE OF CONTENTS

Medical Steps

Information Steps

Treatment Steps

Physical Steps

Waiting Steps

Emotional Steps

Relationship Steps

Steps You Wanted to Know About but Were Afraid to Ask

Appendices

ACKNOWLEDGMENTS

Thank you to my close circle of dearest friends and loved ones who encouraged me to keep writing about my husband Bryan's cancer journey. You did it! You forwarded my e-mail updates to other families dealing with cancer, until our small intimate group expanded to hundreds and hundreds of us holding hands and comparing notes through our cancer journeys. You're the greatest!

Thank you to my many friends who shared your varied experiences with cancer, either as a patient or as a caregiver. Your insights, thoughts, and medical choices have added depth to this book and made my family's journey more bearable. Please e-mail me (and share with others) your cancer journey updates or stop in to chat online at *www.SteppingThroughCancer.com* and *SteppingThroughCancer.blogspot.com*!

Thanks to Dr. Joanne Ruch, my friend and medical adviser, for taking the time to verify the medical information provided in this book.

Thanks also to Dr. Steven Kallick, Bryan's oncologist, who reviewed my manuscript and made sure I covered all the steps.

Thank you to Virelle Kidder, an amazing writer and speaker, who suggested I turn my personal experience into a step-by-step help book for those traveling this road. She saw this book as a possibility after reading only one chapter of my personal experience.

Thanks to fellow authors with the Brighton Writers' Critique Group for painstakingly reading paragraph after paragraph and giving constructive criticism.

Many, many thanks to my friend Polly Flaim for taking the time to edit the final draft for me and reading the entire book twice!

Special thanks to my new friend and fellow author, C. Hope Flinchbaugh, for her great ideas and wonderful editing suggestions. She could see the help and encouragement in this book and on my face. Her website is *www.SeeHope.com*.

Since Bryan didn't go through all these steps in his cancer journey, I did research online and in print. Thanks to the American Cancer Society, the National Cancer Institute, and other cancer organizations for their detailed

information. Their websites and many others have pages and pages of information, too much for someone in the midst of cancer to digest.

I tried to take all the information I found and distill it down to a few pages
for each step that a patient or caregiver could understand. I am grateful for
every source provided and for all their free advice available to anyone with
access to a computer.

Special thanks to Steven Curtis Chapman and Matt Bronleewe for
permission to quote their lyrics.[1]

[1] Lyrics to "The Miracle Of The Moment" used by permission:
The Miracle Of The Moment
Words and Music by Steven Curtis Chapman and Matt Bronleewe
© 2007 SPARROW SONG (BMI), PRIMARY WAVE BRIAN (CHAPMAN
SP ACCT) (BMI), BUG MUSIC-MUSIC OF WINDSWEPT (ASCAP) and
WOODLAND CREATURES NEED MUSIC TOO (ASCAP)
SPARROW SONG Admin. at EMICMGPUBLISHING.COM
All Rights for WOODLAND CREATURES NEED MUSIC TOO Administered
by BUG MUSIC-MUSIC OF WINDSWEPT
All Rights Reserved Used by Permission.

INTRODUCTION

A Few Notes About This Book

- **This is not a medical reference book and was not written by a medical professional.** It was written by a caregiver to educate you about the process and offer practical ideas to make your life easier. **It is not intended to take the place of professional medical help or advice.**

- This book is not intended to be read from cover to cover. Read only the section(s) you need for what you're facing today.

- If you have time to read only one section, read "Medical Step 1—We just got the diagnosis. Now what?" This will give you a few simple ideas to help you care for your loved one.

- The steps are not in chronological order. They are numbered only for convenience. Chemotherapy and radiation are common treatments for cancer, but they don't appear in this book until the Treatment Steps.

- There are suggestions for patients and caregivers as well as family and friends. See the Appendices at the end of the book for specific hints.

- When talking about the patient, they are referred to as "the patient" and "your loved one," assuming that you are caring for someone you love. It helps to remember that you love this person. You may hate the cancer and what it has done to your loved one, but you still love him or her. Let them know!

- Many of these ideas are just common sense. However, when you're facing cancer, common sense is neither common nor sensible.

- Some suggestions appear in more than one step as they apply.

- Not everyone will go through every step listed. Don't think that because you're fighting cancer, you'll face everything in this book. We didn't. Every case is different.

- Fight the cancer each step of the way. This book will give you some ammunition for the battle.

MEDICAL STEPS

MEDICAL STEP 1—WE JUST GOT THE DIAGNOSIS. NOW WHAT?

Your loved one has cancer. Very few words in the English language can have an effect on a person like that phrase.

Your loved one has cancer. It affects not only the patient but also family members and friends.

Your loved one has cancer. A sense of "normal" will come again. For now, wait.

Your loved one has cancer.

Others cannot understand your shock unless they've been there. If you are with the patient as the news is delivered, you just hold hands or hold each other. Everything around you gets quiet and blurred as you try to get your head around it. You can't grasp the concept no matter how hard you try. You sit quietly, not knowing what to say. You know that if you open your mouth, out will come uncontrollable sobs, not words.

When we got the news of my husband's cancer, we sat in the hospital room for half an hour, hands intertwined, tears finding their way down our cheeks. We whispered a little to each other, but I have no memory what we said. I think the word "wow" was softly spoken because of the shock, but we didn't know enough to even discuss the cancer. All we knew was that cancer was there and we'd find out later how we could fight it. No fighting now, just astonishment.

More questions than answers

There are more questions right now than answers.

- What kind of cancer does my loved one have?
- How bad is it?
- How long has it been there?
- How soon can you take it out?
- How will we treat it?
- How can this be?

- What do we do now?
- Who else do we need to talk to?
- Can we get a second opinion? Maybe it's not cancer.

There's no need to answer these questions right away. Time and experience will provide the answers.

Slow down. Write it down. Sit down.

There are three things you can do now to give you some control in the journey:

- Slow down.
- Write it down.
- Sit down.

Slow Down

Take your time doing everything. No matter how fast you normally do things, don't hurry now. You will realize that rushing is hard to do right now, whether walking, talking, driving, or whatever. You'll need to concentrate more than ever to avoid accidents on the road or in the kitchen.

My brain refused to let me work as fast as normal. I had to concentrate just to make coffee, or I'd forget to put water in the coffee maker before I pressed Start. When clearing the table, if I didn't pay attention, the milk would end up in the cupboard and the oatmeal box in the refrigerator. I had to stop and think before I did anything, and make myself conscious of even little things.

Take your time doing everything, even speaking. You may say something you'll regret if you just blurt things out, especially to those closest to you, including the patient. It's better if you bite your tongue and don't say something that may hurt. Once said, it can't be unsaid. Just take a deep breath.

Write It Down

Write down things that you don't want to forget. Write down:

- Everything the doctor tells you.
- The name of the cancer, and ask for the spelling if you need it.

- Questions that come to mind. You can ask them at a later appointment. Just write down the questions.
- Any feelings you have. These will come in waves and extremes. Don't think about your feelings. Just feel them and write them down.
- People you need to call. You can look up their phone numbers later. Just write down their names.
- Whatever you need to do right away, like cancel the babysitter tonight or reschedule the plumber for next week. Just write it down as you think of it.
- Things that you planned on doing "someday," and make plans to do them. It will give you a few moments of hope and escape. If you do have the opportunity to fulfill one of your dreams, don't put it off. Do it! But for now, write them down.

Writing down everything is the only way to remember, because you won't be able to rely on your brain for a while. Don't beat yourself up over it; that's just the way it is. No one will be upset or disappointed that you're human. Your life just came crashing down, and what used to be normal will never be normal again.

When Bryan was diagnosed, we decided to watch the movie "The Bucket List," starring Jack Nicholson and Morgan Freeman. It's about two senior citizens who decide to accomplish some of the things they had planned to do before they died. Bryan and I created our own Bucket List, things that we would do when Bryan's cancer went into remission. It gave us something else to think about, happy memories that we planned to create, and a momentary lapse of reality when we needed it.

Sit Down

Don't try to do everything you usually do. Take time to just sit, think, and talk with those who love you. Right now, you just need to *be* ... just be. Your mind is having a hard time digesting the news, so don't push it. The battle ahead is the most important thing in your life right now.

You also will be doing a lot of waiting: for doctor's appointments, in the emergency room, and for pending test results. You may as well get used to it.

This may be the time to make sure your finances are organized. Bryan had always handled our bills and payments, so he took the time to show me where he had budget information and receipts. Since I would be paying the bills while he was fighting cancer, it helped me to know where everything was located.

Here are a few more suggestions to help you through the journey:

- Put things away in the same place every time. It's easy to just drop things when you're done with them, like most people do all the time, but you may not remember where you left them.

Keep your keys handy and the gas tank full.

- You *must* find your car keys in a hurry if you need to go to the emergency room. Spending time looking for them is not an option. You may want to put a hook inside the door and hang them up every time you come home, so they'll be visible and handy the next time you need them. Also, put your purse or wallet nearby so you can grab it on the way out.
- Keep your car's gas tank full in case you need to leave in a hurry.
- Let others know what you're going through. Read "Relationship Step 1—Who do we tell? And how?" for specific ideas. You'd be surprised how many people care and want to help you.
- Don't be afraid to ask for help. "Relationship Step 5—Asking for and receiving help" will show you how and when to ask, and how to accept help. This may relieve you of some tasks, such as keeping the house clean or the lawn mowed. Offer loved ones the gift of helping you.
- One of the most useful things you can do now is to stay organized. Your life feels out of control, and knowing where things are is the first step to being in control. Don't try to organize your closets or dresser drawers; that would be too much to tackle. Just keep all your info and paperwork on cancer in one location so they're easier to find. And putting things away will make your life less cluttered in more ways than one.
- Do small, mindless tasks that you can control. One caregiver took this opportunity to alphabetize her spices, something that she could handle without help.

Prepare a tote bag.

Get a bag ready to take to appointments or the emergency room, which you may find yourself visiting frequently. It's better to prepare now rather than as you're running out the door, trying to remember what you need to take.

Here is a list of things to put in a tote bag and keep by the door:

- The patient's health care identification card and photo ID. Most health care providers will not give any medical care unless you have a valid health care ID and a photo ID such as a driver's license.
- A list of the patient's medications and doses.
- A list of contacts and telephone numbers. Include your doctors as well as family, close friends, and your pastor or other religious leader. This is easier to carry than a Rolodex or a Day-Timer, and quicker than a cell phone.
- Cell phone charger. You can dig it out if you need it at home.
- A sweater. Since bacteria grow more slowly in a cooler temperature, hospitals keep the rooms uncomfortably cold. The patient can get blankets, but the caregiver generally cannot.
- A note pad and pen to write down everything that happens. If you have a notebook as explained in "Information Step 1— What do I do with all the paperwork and information we get?" keep that in the tote bag.
- A water bottle for the caregiver.
- An energy bar or other snacks.
- Magazine, book, or crossword/Sudoku books and pen to pass the time.
- Some cash, in case you need to buy snacks or a meal from a vending machine while you're waiting.

Your life has just changed dramatically. Take your time getting used to the idea and adjusting. You've just started a journey that many others have taken or are in the midst of. You can manage your journey one step at a time.

MEDICAL STEP 2—MEETING WITH THE ONCOLOGIST

Oncologist means "cancer doctor" or "cancer specialist," someone who studies, diagnoses, and treats cancerous tumors. I will use the masculine "he" for the oncologist, since ours was a man.

Write everything down.

The number one thing when meeting with the oncologist is to write everything down. I guarantee you won't remember everything he says, especially if you're emotional. And anything you might remember could be different from what was actually said. You can take a small digital recorder to appointments, but be sure to put it down on paper later, so you can find the info when you need it.

At least two people at every appointment.

The second most important thing is to be sure there are at least two people in the room for every appointment: the patient and one other. If the "one other" is not good at taking notes, have a third person there to write everything down. The doctor won't mind and will be glad that someone is keeping track of what is said, as it will cut down on questions later. Also, your family members are less likely to argue with what you wrote than with what you just remember from the visit.

Our oncologist, Dr. Steven Kallick, entered the room, introduced himself, shook our hands warmly, and then pulled up a chair. This indicated that he was there to talk with us for as long as necessary, not to just talk and leave. He was very sensitive to our concerns, taking the time to give us the name of the cancer, spell it for me to write it down, and explain where it was, how it got there, and how it might be treated. He even apologized for giving us bad news.

If your oncologist is not compassionate, ask for a different doctor. This cancer is now the most important thing in your life, and you need to feel that the oncologist is on your team and fighting with you, not clinical and standing on the side watching you two fight alone. He should take the time you need to explain the situation and options for treatment.

Write down questions to ask.

As a specialist, your oncologist will have more knowledge of the cancer than anyone else you'll meet in this journey. Take advantage of that resource. I'm not telling you to call him any hour of the day or night, but if you think of a question to ask, write it down and take it to the next appointment. No question is too small, too complex, or too dumb for your oncologist. He would rather have a patient and caregiver working with him and following his advice to the letter than forgetting his advice and waiting for whatever may come next. That would be a waste of everyone's time.

If possible, get a second and possibly a third opinion. This is literally a life-or-death situation, and you have every right to ask another specialist. Your oncologist should not be threatened by your desire for another analysis. In fact, most doctors welcome it. The two (or three) doctors can confer on their diagnoses and suggested treatments, which will result in a better outcome. After all, two heads are better than one.

MEDICAL STEP 3—WHAT'S A CT OR CAT SCAN?

CT stands for Computed Tomography. It can also be called a CAT scan, which stands for Computerized Axial Tomography. It's basically another form of x-ray. The main difference is that while an x-ray is a two-dimensional picture, a CT is three-dimensional.

For a CT, many two-dimensional pictures are taken of the inside of the patient while the camera rotates around an axis. Then, the pictures are all put together to create the three-dimensional image. My friend Dr. Joanne Ruch describes CT images to her patients as "slices of the body, like a sliced ham."

A CT scan is used when a doctor needs to see all sides of a tumor, to determine its size, and to find out if it has spread. It gives a much more realistic picture of what you are facing.

Allergic to iodine?

Sometimes an iodine dye is injected to give a clearer picture. Be sure to tell your doctor if the patient is allergic to iodine or any other medicines. This can be injected through an IV in the arm, directly into the spinal cord, or sometimes taken orally. Ask the doctor or technician how it will be administered. If the patient has any hesitation about the method, ask if there is an alternative. Be sure to have your loved one drink lots of liquids for 24 hours after the procedure to help flush the dye out of the body.

A patient may have a reaction to the dye, but this is rare and is usually just itching or hives. If there is difficulty breathing, notify medical personnel immediately, as this may be life-threatening. Let your doctor know of any reaction. There may be a simple over-the-counter or home remedy to help.

The CT itself is painless and can take from 30 to 90 minutes. The patient is placed on a movable table which slides into the center of a large, donut-shaped machine. It is important for the patient to remain as still and quiet as possible during the CT scan procedure to get clear pictures. The technologist tells the patient when to breathe or hold his or her breath during scans of the chest and abdomen. The technologist will observe through a window and use an intercom to talk with the patient.

The CT scanner is basically a tube that you lie inside, so let the doctor know if the patient tends to become nervous in small spaces. He can sedate the patient for the procedure. Be sure someone drives the patient home afterward if a sedative is used.

The amount of radiation received during a CT scan is minimal, and normally does not produce any side effects. If a pregnant woman needs a CT scan, let the doctor know her condition. An ultrasound is a safer alternative for the unborn baby.

MEDICAL STEP 4—WHAT'S A PET SCAN?

PET stands for Positron Emission Tomography. This is a nuclear imaging technique that produces a three-dimensional picture similar to a CT scan but with much broader images. Not only does a PET scan help in diagnosing, but it can also eliminate unnecessary surgery and indicate how a tumor is responding to chemotherapy. Some newer machines are able to perform both a PET scan and a CT scan at the same time, saving you one extra appointment.

PET stands for Positron Emission Tomography.

For a PET scan, a form of sugar (glucose) with a trace of radioactivity is injected by IV into a vein. Within 30 minutes, the cancer attracts the sugar into its cells, which can then be photographed by the computer/camera. Any cancer cells appear as black spots.

The injection may give the patient an overall warm feeling. This is natural and not harmful. A female friend was warned before her PET scan that the injection in women may make them feel that they have to go to the bathroom. Ask the technician if this might happen and what he or she would like the patient to do, as the procedure may take some time.

Take a book for the wait.

Because of the radioactivity and the x-ray-type machine, the patient will be alone in the room during the procedure, which lasts from 30 minutes to an hour, although the technician is on an intercom. The caregiver may want to take a book or something to pass the time while waiting.

A PET scan is very expensive procedure and is not equally effective in all cancers, so some health care organizations may not want to pay for it. Your oncologist will determine if a PET scan would be beneficial for your loved one.

When checking in for the procedure, ask if they will give you a CD of the results. It may take a few minutes after the procedure is done, but it's worth the wait, and usually at minimal or no cost. You can see a three-dimensional image of the entire body, which rotates so you can see it from all sides. Any tumors will show up as black spots. The doctor may not call with results for a few days, so you can view the CD on your own. This may or may not be a good idea, but it's up to you and the patient.

There is so little radioactivity injected, it will probably not create any side effects. However, if the patient has trouble breathing, get medical help immediately.

Just as with a CT scan, have the patient drink plenty of fluids in the next 24 hours to rid the body of the radioactivity.

MEDICAL STEP 5—HAVING A PORT (CATHETER) OR STENT INSERTED

There are times when the human body needs help in keeping passages open for such things as liver draining, infusing chemotherapy, or frequent blood draws without getting needle-poked every time. This can be accomplished easily by inserting a stent to keep a passage wide enough to function correctly, or a port to give medical personnel easy access during procedures.

A stent is a small, mesh tube inserted internally into a duct or artery to keep fluids flowing. It is commonly used for angioplasty to keep arteries around the heart open. It can also be used in bile ducts to allow the liver to drain toxins from the body, which is its normal function. The liver must process all the poisons from chemotherapy and get rid of them, so it needs to drain properly.

A stent is internal. A port is external.

When a stent is inserted into a bile duct, the patient "swallows" a tube containing the stent, and the doctor sets the stent in place. Then, the tube is carefully removed. The process is somewhat uncomfortable but is a necessary step for the body to get rid of all the poison. The stent will need to be replaced about every three months for the rest of the patient's life, even if they beat the cancer, unless the bile duct starts to drain on its own. Removing the stent also involves "swallowing" a tube.

A port, sometimes called a catheter, is a thin plastic tube inserted into the body for any of a number of reasons. Bryan's doctors called it a catheter, but my medical expert says it's usually called a port. A small port may be inserted into a vein in the patient's forearm or hand (an IV) at each chemotherapy treatment for the chemicals to flow into the veins. In cases where the patient's veins are tired of all the poking, a port can be inserted into the chest cavity to avoid the need for an IV to be inserted at every chemo treatment. It will remain in place for the duration of treatment, not just for the day. Blood can also be drawn through the port, avoiding another poke with a needle.

For liver drainage, a catheter is inserted through the abdomen into the liver so it can drain outside the body. This may be necessary when the cancer is blocking the bile ducts, as was the case for us. The blockage was evident by the jaundiced (yellow) appearance of Bryan's skin and eyes. Within hours of the catheter insertion, Bryan's color was returning to normal and he felt much better.

The catheter is left in the body and taped in place so it will not move. A bag is attached to the tube, and may have a strap to wrap around the patient's waist and keep it in place.

The bag of bile can be emptied easily. If physically able, the patient can empty the bag into the toilet while sitting on "the throne" so it can be simply flushed away. If not, the caretaker will need to empty it into a container, then dump it into the toilet and wash the container with soap and water. There is a very unpleasant odor to the bile, so don't stand directly above where you're draining. I guarantee you'll only do it once!

In time, the catheter may start to work itself out of the body, so you'll notice more of the tube outside the body. This is normal, but let your doctor know. He may choose to leave it, or remove it and insert another catheter.

Follow your health care provider's instructions for cleaning and maintaining the port or catheter. It is a permanent, non-healing opening into your loved one's body and you don't want any bacteria or contaminants entering through it, making your loved one even sicker.

MEDICAL STEP 6—WHAT IS REMISSION? DOES IT MEAN CANCER-FREE?

Often, remission is thought to mean that the cancer is gone. While this might hopefully be the case, many times remission means the cancer is responding to treatment or is under control. Any symptoms are now more bearable or are completely gone.

There are two types of remission: complete and partial.

Complete remission means no cancer is detected.

Complete Remission

In complete remission, cancer cannot be detected by any available tests, and all symptoms and signs of cancer disappear. Life can go back to a "new normal" with no more cancer treatments. However, since there is a chance that cancer may recur in the same place or elsewhere in the body, your oncologist will conduct regular checkups to detect any new growths.

Early detection is always a plus in cancer treatment, so keeping all oncology appointments will give the patient and the doctor an advantage in case of recurrence. Even if all tests show no signs of cancer, it is wise to get checked as often as the oncologist recommends.

Partial remission means the tumor shrank.

Partial Remission

In partial remission, there is a noticeable decrease in cancer cells (the tumor has shrunk), and only a few remaining symptoms and signs of cancer. The oncologist may recommend continued treatment as long as it is beneficial. If treatment does more harm than good, such as when the side effects are getting worse, the doctor may suggest delaying additional treatment.

Whatever is recommended, be sure you and the patient are comfortable with it. If the patient wants to continue treatment and can bear the side effects, ask the oncologist if there is a good chance that it will make a difference in the fight. The doctor will make recommendations, but it is up to the patient what treatments to pursue. As the caregiver, you need to be in agreement so you can support your loved one. Be sure you agree with any decision.

MEDICAL STEP 7—HOW LONG DOES REMISSION LAST?

Remission, both partial and complete, can last for weeks, months, or years. A complete remission that lasts for years is often considered a cure.

My younger brother, Ken, had cancer in his early twenties. It had spread to multiple locations in his body with some tumors as large as an orange. After surgery, chemotherapy, and radiation, his cancer went into complete remission. Ken turned 56 this year, with no recurrence of cancer. I have two other friends who had breast cancer 17 and 30 years ago and have been in complete remission since then.

What to do during remission? LIVE!

What do you do during remission? Live! Live life to the fullest. Most people have no idea how precious life is, but you know it first-hand. Now is the chance for your loved one to do all those things that have been put off, those things on his or her Bucket List. Take the time to visit family, travel, write, paint, sing, dance, and do all those things you couldn't during the cancer fight. Enjoy life!

Regular checkups give the doctor a chance to detect any new cancer early, which increases the chance of successful treatment. Should the cancer come back, the new cancer can be in any part of the body. It may respond to a different treatment, such as a different drug combination or radiation instead of surgery, which the oncologist will determine. Treatment can lead to another remission, which is another lease on life.

Multiple remissions are common, so don't give up if the cancer comes back. It's a new opportunity for you and your loved one, a speed bump in the road of life. Look at this new fight as a step toward another remission.

Don't give up!

MEDICAL STEP 8—THE CANCER HAS COME BACK. NOW WHAT?

"Your cancer has come back." That's one of the most heartbreaking sentences you could ever hear. After the first diagnosis of cancer and the time and energy it took to fight it, remission was the rest that you and your loved one needed so desperately. During remission, it was great not having that black cloud hanging over you all the time.

Now your lives have come crashing down again. You and your loved one may have tried to ignore the symptoms that were creeping up, but they were unmistakably there. Your oncologist has just given you the news. Where do you go from here?

You both may feel angry, sad, scared, hopeless, shocked, or a myriad of other emotions. That's normal. But feelings are just that—feelings. So be aware of them as they come and then get on with your cancer fight.

Some people may think they don't have the emotional or physical ability to handle another round of treatments. However, attitude is a major factor in the success of treatment. Learn as much as you can about this new cancer. Knowledge will help the patient, the caregiver, and any medical professional involved in the treatment. Make up your mind that since you won the last round, you can and will win this one as well. Help your loved one to be of the same mind.

Advantages to recurrence

There are several advantages now that you didn't have when you heard the first diagnosis.

- Experience. You know the steps needed, the treatments and their side effects, and that gives you a head start in the fight.
- Medical treatment is continually improving. Drugs available now may not have been around the first time you were fighting. Those drugs can do a better job of treating the cancer

and minimizing side effects, so this go-round may be easier than before.

- You and the patient have a relationship with the oncologist and other medical professionals, so you won't be meeting with strangers like the first time. There may be some new people, but chances are you'll know some of the doctors, technicians, and nurses, not to mention other patients and caregivers undergoing treatment along with you.

Communication is key in any cancer fight. Tell the doctor what the patient feels and what side effects he or she has. Let him know if your loved one needs any help that you can't provide, such as daily tasks, sleeping, or managing pain or nausea. Keeping the patient's body as strong as possible will help in the fight.

Keep a positive attitude.

A positive attitude will go miles toward a success. The patient will draw emotions from those around him or her, so don't be negative in his or her presence. Encouragement is vital in this battle. The doctor isn't giving up, so neither should anyone else.

INFORMATION STEPS

INFORMATION STEP 1—WHAT DO I DO WITH ALL THE PAPERWORK AND INFORMATION WE GET?

Beginning with the first doctor's appointment, you will be given more information than you can ever hope to absorb. In addition to the receipt, the self-care instructions, and so on that you receive after the initial visit, you will be bombarded with paper, verbal facts and figures, instructions for referrals, and a ton of other data. Organizing these as soon as possible will help you to use the info. Maybe you can't make sense of the cancer, but you can make sense of all the information you have.

My friend Dr. Joanne Ruch suggests that her patients get a three-ring notebook to hold all the papers. A two-inch size with pockets is good to start with.

Create a handbook/notebook.

Use tabbed dividers for the following sections:

- Personal Phone List (group them by type, such as family, work, medical).
- Notes (that you take at appointments and treatments).
- Questions (to ask the doctor).
- Prescriptions and Other Medications.
- Medical info (from the web or handouts from your doctor).
- Results.
- Encouragement (e-mails or cards you receive).
- Insurance.
- Bills, Financial Statements, and related Correspondence.
- Planning for the Future (plans for the future, or a Bucket List).
- Peace of Mind – Taking Control.
- Hospice (if you need it).
- Misc. info (anything that doesn't fit in the sections above).

It's OK to punch holes in all the papers you'll be inserting. Nothing in your book will lose its value just because it has a few holes in it.

Personal Phone List is for a list of everyone you may need to call for any reason. You won't need to call everyone in your family, but be sure you have someone who will relay information if needed. As you have time, look up their numbers (home, work, and cell) and write them here. Don't rely on your cell phone, as the battery may die while you spend time in an ER or a hospital room. It's much easier if you have all the phone numbers written and in one place.

Notes will be where you write down everything. Put in 20-30 pages of lined notebook paper, not the college size. You want to be able to write large and be able to read it later. Write down weight, temperature, and blood pressure at every doctor visit, whether a scheduled appointment or a visit to the emergency room. You'll be surprised how often you need to refer back to see what the stats were previously.

Write down everything a doctor or nurse tells you, no matter how unimportant you may feel it is. Right now, you can't think straight, so something you might deem trivial may be something that you'll need in the near future.

This section will also contain printouts your doctor may give you after an appointment. These normally include the same stats you just wrote, but will also contain instructions to follow between visits. Keep them handy, because you'll need to refer to them often.

Questions will contain 5-10 pages of lined notebook paper, again not college size. Whenever you think of a question to ask the doctor, write it here. Leave a few lines between questions for you to write the answers. When you're visiting the doctor, you'll be able to ask all those questions that you thought you wouldn't forget but did. Write down the answers as you get them; don't rely on your memory.

Prescriptions and Other Medications is for all the paperwork you get about any medication your loved one is taking or may take. This will include prescriptions and any other over-the-counter or other medication. You may also do some online research which you'll want to keep here. Don't rely on your memory for dosage or interaction info. Keep it here for easy reference.

Medical Info is where you put all the information you receive about cancer, this specific cancer, treatment, nutrition, or any other facts you receive. As you search the web for information and print pages of interest, insert them here.

Results is for any test results you receive on paper. This will provide a place that's easy to find if you need to refer back to anything. You can then also see any progress the treatment has made.

Encouragement is for printed e-mails that you or your loved one receives with positive support, printed web pages that you come across that you'd like to read again and again, and any other documents that give you hope. Don't try to insert all the cards you receive, as the notebook may become too large. If you get a few with messages that you want to read again and again, put them into sheet protectors and put them here.

Insurance is for any paperwork you get involving insurance. This may be statements of coverage, bills, or correspondence.

Bills, Financial Statements, and Related Correspondence will contain all the statements you receive from the doctor, hospital, or pharmacy, as well as any letters about them. You may want to ask a family member or trusted friend who is not so emotionally connected to review the bills for accuracy.

Planning for the Future can also be called **Hope**. This section will have 1-2 sheets of notebook paper for you and your loved ones to make a "bucket list" of things that you still want to do, especially when this cancer goes into remission. List big things like vacations you want to take and little things like the ice cream flavor you want to try. Besides giving you a quick reference when you have the ability to fulfill a dream, it will give you a minute to escape reality as you dream about the future.

Peace of Mind – Taking Control is for advance directives, which everyone should have in place, not just cancer patients. Be sure your family knows how your loved one wants to be treated, so their wishes are followed.

Hospice information is an optional section. Most cancer patients won't need this section, so don't add it unless you do.

Misc. Info is for anything that doesn't fit into another section. You'll receive more data than you think you'll ever need, so just put it here. Then you'll be able find it if and when you need it.

If you think of any other sections, feel free to add them. You may want one for recipes or for information on treatment centers. Add whatever you need to keep handy.

Create a notebook for a friend.

You may want to create a blank notebook for a friend or loved one when he or she receives the cancer diagnosis. They will thank you many times over.

INFORMATION STEP 2—WHERE CAN I FIND MORE INFORMATION?

There are many resources to tap for information:

- Your doctor or health care provider.
- The web.
- Your local library.
- A bookstore.

Write down questions for your doctor.

Your Doctor or Health Care Provider

Your doctor or health care provider will be glad to provide you with as much information as you can carry. Don't hesitate to ask at any appointment. They will likely have some brochures or handouts to explain treatments, tests, procedures, possible side effects, and a myriad of other things the patient may encounter on the journey.

The Web

The World Wide Web will give over 70 million results when you search for "cancer." Since anyone can create a website and put anything on it that they want, you'll need to sort out the good information from the bad.

Try to stay with the "safe" sites, such as renowned medical sites and government sites with a URL that ends in .gov. These have a reputation to maintain and will have more accurate info.

Here are some reputable websites:

- American Cancer Society at *www.cancer.org.*
- National Institutes of Health, which lists itself as "The Nation's Medical Research Agency" at *www.nih.gov* lists 27 different health entities, including:
  - o National Cancer Institute at *www.cancer.gov.*
  - o National Center for Complementary and Alternative Medicine at *www.nccam.nih.gov.*
  - o National Library of Medicine at *nlm.nih.gov.*
  - o Many others that may have information on cancer.
- MedicineNet.com at *www.medicinenet.com* states that it complies with the HON (Health On the Net Foundation) code standard for trustworthy health information.
- WebMD at *www.webmd.com* has the same HON code.

You can also check online dictionaries and encyclopedias, such as the National Library of Medicine at *www.nlm.nih.gov*, Answers at *www. answers.com*, or Merriam-Webster Online at *www.merriam-webster.com/ dictionary/cancer*. Some people enjoy reading what is posted on the encyclopedia of the people—Wikipedia. If that's you, please go to Wikipedia at *www.en.wikipedia.org.*

Don't try to research every topic for every type of cancer.

Some cancer societies are for mainly one type of cancer and don't try to cover every topic for every type of cancer. You may find those websites are more specific to your needs.

When in doubt about the validity of the information, scroll to the bottom of the home page and see who sponsors the website. Many are sponsored by a drug company, just out to push their cure for whatever ails you, or a special treatment center, out to get your health care dollars.

Even something innocuous or medical-sounding can be a drug company's advertising page. Be sure to verify the source.

Your Local Library

You can look through the card catalog of your local library on your home computer. You may find your library or extended library system has books, reference books, and magazines with information. Be sure to find publications with a recent copyright or published date, since medical advances happen every day. Note that reference books and magazines must not leave the library, so have either paper and pen to take notes or cash for printing applicable pages to take with you.

A Bookstore

Your local bookstore will have books on cancer in their health section. Unfortunately, I've found them to be on the bottom shelf of the women's health section. Apparently there aren't enough books on cancer yet to warrant their own section. You can always ask a salesperson for help in locating them.

Some of the books available are written by medical professionals and cover every type of cancer there is, so you may find a 1,000-page book with only a few pages on the type of cancer you're dealing with. If possible, take the time to peruse all the available books so you get the ones that will do you the most good.

Don't expect to understand everything you read. In fact, you may not understand anything at all. This is normal. Your brain is under stress right now, so it's not working as well as usual. When my friends brought books during Bryan's illness, I could read ten pages and not remember a thing I read.

Feel free to highlight things you want to remember (unless it's a library or loaned book) or write them in your notebook, so you can refer back to them when needed. Also, these may trigger some questions that you want to ask the doctor at the next appointment. Write these questions in your notebook.

INFORMATION STEP 3—HOW CAN
I KEEP TABS ON THE DOCTORS,
NURSES, AND MEDICATIONS?

The most effective way to keep track of everything is to write it all down. You'll find that it helps to have it in writing, especially when your brain is preoccupied with fighting cancer.

> **Write down the doctor's answers during your appointment.**

If a doctor or nurse sees that you're recording everything they say, they'll be sure that you understand completely. My experience is that they will tell you more if they sense that you're really paying attention.

Several friends mentioned that when their loved ones were in the hospital, they would make a surprise visit at any hour of the day or night. It was an eye-opener to drop in at 2 A.M. and see what was happening.

One friend just happened to be in the room when a nurse was about to take her father's blood pressure in an arm that contained a stent. Even though there was a sign on the door indicating blood pressure was only to be taken in the right arm, the nurse placed the cuff on the left arm. Anyone can make a mistake, so being able to protect your loved one from such a problem is important. Be aware of restrictions, and make sure all instructions are followed to the letter.

Most doctors will give you a business card with their information on it. Keep those handy. You may also find it helpful to create a list of all your contacts, both medical and personal, and keep it with you when you go for appointments or treatments. It will help to have it on paper in case your cell phone battery dies.

You may want to create a list of all caregivers, including nurses and aides, and write down the dates you see them. This is easy to do in a spreadsheet program on the computer or on a piece of paper with columns.

Just write their names in the first column, their titles in the second column, and the dates in the rest of the columns. You'll also see at a glance when and how often you saw each person.

When you take notes at each visit, it'll be easy to cross-reference those notes with this list. That way, if you have a particular question about something that was said at an appointment, you'll know who to ask for clarification.

Keep an ongoing list of meds and their side effects.

Keeping a list of medications, dosages, and the times they were given will help the doctor or nurse when treating side effects. If a symptom started after taking a high dosage of a certain medication, the dosage may be lowered to reduce the side effects. Or if meds counteract each other, the health professionals will know to spread them out.

Create a list in a spreadsheet or on notebook paper. List each medication and next to it write the date, time, and dosage. Or you may want to just list the time the meds are given and write out each drug and dosage. Either way, keeping track of when medications are taken will benefit both patient and doctor.

INFORMATION STEP 4—
WHAT DO WE TAKE WITH US TO
THE EMERGENCY ROOM?

You may find yourself rushing to the emergency room many times on your loved one's cancer journey. It's best if you prepare for it so you won't take too long gathering things or forget anything necessary.

Prepare a tote bag.

Get a tote bag, briefcase, or something large enough to hold your loose-leaf notebook plus a few other things. You don't need to spend any money—just find a bag around the house.

Here are some items to put in your tote bag and keep by the door:

- The patient's health care identification card and photo ID. Most health care providers will not give any medical care unless you have a valid health care ID and a photo ID such as a driver's license.
- A list of the patient's medications and doses.
- A list of contacts and telephone numbers. Include your doctors as well as family, close friends, and your pastor or other religious leader. This is easier to carry than a Rolodex or a Day-Timer, and quicker than a cell phone.
- Cell phone charger. You can dig it out if you need it at home.
- A sweater. Since bacteria grow more slowly in a cooler temperature, hospitals keep the rooms uncomfortably cold. The patient can get blankets, but the caregiver often cannot.
- A note pad and pen to write down everything that happens. If you have a notebook as explained in "Information Step 1— What do I do with all the paperwork and information we get?" keep that in the tote bag.
- A water bottle for the caregiver.
- An energy bar or other snacks.

- Magazine, book, or crossword/Sudoku books and pen to pass the time.
- Some cash, in case you need to buy snacks or a meal from a vending machine while you're waiting.

Keep your keys handy and the gas tank full.

Keep your car keys and purse or wallet near the door, so you can pick them up on your way out. You don't want to waste precious time trying to find them when you need to get on the road.

Also, keep your car's gas tank full. If the gas gauge gets down to one-fourth, fill the tank on your way home. You don't want to waste time stopping at a gas station on your way to the ER.

Be prepared to spend time in the emergency room. In addition to the number of patients to be seen, you may need to wait for test results, x-rays, CT scans, or any number of medical procedures. You can't rush them, so everyone needs to be patient. Maybe that's where they got the word "patient."

If you feel you will need to make a trip to the ER, don't wait until evening or night if possible. That's when ERs get busy, and you'll have a longer wait. Go when you must, but realize that you may spend more time there in the evening.

TREATMENT STEPS

TREATMENT STEP 1— WILL SURGERY HELP?

Surgery is the oldest form of cancer treatment. It is also useful in diagnosing cancer and determining how far it has spread. Newer surgical techniques allow doctors to remove cancers with less cutting and damage to nearby tissues or organs.

Most people with cancer will have some type of surgery. A minor surgery is called a procedure. This can involve inserting a stent or a catheter, or any number of other procedures.

Preventive Surgery

Preventive surgery can be performed to remove an organ from a patient with an inherited condition that puts them at higher risk of having cancer some day. This could be for a woman whose family has a history of breast cancer and whose DNA of the cancer gene has mutated. Removing breasts before cancer is found may eliminate the possibility of cancer and its potential to spread to any other organs.

Diagnostic Surgery

Surgery can also be done for diagnostic reasons. The doctor will take a sample of tissue to see if cancer is present by examining it under a microscope. This can be accomplished through an incision, or by inserting a fine needle into the tumor and withdrawing some cells without an incision and the recovery period that would require.

Determining the stage of cancer can also be accomplished through surgery. This will help the doctor to see how much cancer there is and how far it has spread. The results will determine a plan of treatment and the prognosis for the patient.

Curative Surgery

In some cases, surgery is the only treatment necessary to totally get rid of cancer. This is called "curative surgery." Surgery can also be done in conjunction with chemotherapy and radiation treatments.

Endoscopy is a procedure that allows the doctor to see the tumor by inserting a tube with a small viewing lens or video camera and a fiber-optic light. Endoscopes can be passed through natural body openings without any cutting. The patient may be under a general anesthetic, and local numbing will make the procedure less uncomfortable.

Laser surgery involves a highly focused beam of light energy for very precise surgical work, resulting in less cutting and damage. This can be performed during an endoscopy, with the laser performing the surgery inside the body and no external cut.

Your oncologist will consult with a surgeon to decide if your loved one's cancer is operable and what type of surgery is best for this cancer. When in doubt, you can always seek a second or third opinion.

Questions to ask before surgery.

Before agreeing, find out all you can about the surgery and its risks, benefits, and side effects. Here is a list of possible questions to ask. Add to this list if you think of anything else you want to know. Write down the answers you receive:

- Why are you suggesting this surgery?
- How soon would you need to operate?
- What will you be taking out?
- How long with the surgery take?
- What are the chances that it will succeed?
- Do you feel my loved one is healthy enough for the surgery, anesthesia, and after-effects?
- Who will be performing the surgery? Are they certified appropriately?
- How many times have they successfully done something similar?
- Is the surgeon familiar with this type of cancer?
- Should we get donations for possible blood transfusions?

- Will my loved one need reconstructive surgery? If so, can it be done at the same time?
- What possible risks are there?
- How long will my loved one have to stay in the hospital?
- Will there be a lot of pain?
- Will he or she need catheters or drains?
- Will there be scarring? What will it look like?
- What side effects can we expect? How will you treat them?
- What is the expected recovery period for this type of surgery?
- Is there another option besides surgery? What if we don't have the surgery?
- How soon do you need to perform the surgery? Can it wait long enough for a second opinion?

The final decision on surgery belongs to the patient.

Don't forget that the final decision on surgery belongs to the patient. Your doctor will give you recommendations for diagnosis and treatment, but the final choice is up to you and your loved one. Learn as much as possible before making your decision.

TREATMENT STEP 2—WHAT CAN WE EXPECT WITH SURGERY?

Some surgeries can be performed in a doctor's office or clinic. Others require hospitalization. The type and extent of your loved one's surgery as well as his or her overall health will determine where and how the surgery is performed.

Not all surgeries are performed immediately. You may have several weeks to wait, so use that time to educate yourself. If immediate surgery is indicated, the oncologist will tell you. Otherwise, take the time you have to ask questions, talk with others who have been through it, and make yourselves more familiar with the procedure. If your doctor recommends a delay in surgery, it will have no impact on the outcome, so don't worry that waiting will make it worse.

Learn as much as you can about this surgical procedure from your doctor and health care provider. Since they will be responsible for and may be performing the procedure, they would know the most about it and will be glad to share information. By knowing as much as you can, you'll reduce your stress level as well as your loved one's, which will help in the recovery.

Don't worry about something that probably won't happen.

Before surgery, the patient will be asked to sign a consent form. This signature indicates that the doctor has explained why the surgery is necessary, the goal of the surgery, how it will be done, what the benefits are, possible side effects, risks, and other treatment options. This is standard for all surgeries.

Don't be alarmed by the list of risks and side effects. The medical community must list every possible outcome, no matter how small the possibility of it happening. Don't even think about any of those negative outcomes. There's no sense worrying about something that probably won't happen.

The patient may need blood tests, urine tests, x-rays, or other tests done prior to surgery. The doctor will provide instructions, such as when your loved one needs to fast or drink extra water before a test.

It's normal for the patient to be nervous or anxious prior to surgery. Talk to your doctor about it, and he may be able to give your loved one something to help them relax.

Anesthesia

The patient will likely be anesthetized during surgery. This may be a localized or regional anesthetic just for the area being operated on, or a general anesthetic, where the patient is put into a deep sleep. When under general anesthetic, a tube is inserted down the throat to help assist with breathing.

If a local anesthetic is used, the patient may go home the same day. Use of a regional or general anesthetic will require some time in the recovery room while the effects of the drugs wear off. Your loved one may need to stay in the hospital for several days after surgery, especially if a general anesthetic is used.

Pain Medications

The patient will receive pain medications during and after the surgery, and a prescription for other pain meds to take at home. A nurse will ask the patient to number the level of pain from 0 to 10, with 0 meaning no pain and 10 meaning the worst possible pain. Tell your loved one to ask for pain meds if the pain goes above 3. It's harder to reduce a pain level that has gotten out of hand than to keep it low.

Your loved one's throat may also be sore from the breathing tube inserted. Ask the doctor what is recommended. It may not require a prescription; however, eating or drinking something soothing may help.

Follow the doctor's instructions regarding eating and drinking. The digestive tract (stomach and intestines) may take a while to recover from any drugs, so the patient may have trouble digesting and passing food or drink. The patient may be on a clear diet for a while, until he or she has passed gas. Let the doctor know when this happens, as it may be a sign that normal eating can resume.

What To Take Home After Surgery

When ready to go home, be sure the doctor provides you with:

- Instructions to care for the incision at home.
- A prescription for pain.
- A list of activity limits, such as driving or lifting restrictions.
- Diet restriction.
- Names and numbers of who to call with questions or problems.
- Directions for any further treatment, such as physical therapy.
- When to see the doctor again.

Being home alone may be a problem for the patient, so if you must work outside the home, see if your family, friends, or health care team can assist. They may offer to stay with your loved one or provide a nurse or nurse's aide to help.

TREATMENT STEP 3—HOW LONG WILL MY LOVED ONE BE IN THE HOSPITAL?

Some hospital stays are just overnight; some are longer. The reason for the admittance will likely determine how long your loved one will remain. A minor procedure may take only one day; major surgery will require a longer recuperation period.

Always add two days to the estimated hospital stay.

A wise doctor once told us to add two days to the time estimate the doctor gives, and you won't be disappointed. That way, if your loved one is released on the day the doctor guessed, all is well. But if they have to stay longer, it's not unexpected.

Most hospital stays will be for only one or two days. If there is any kind of procedure or surgery, your loved one may need to stay in a recovery room at least until his or her vital signs are normal. That might involve an overnight stay.

Also, if the surgery is more extensive or involved a general anesthesia, the patient will be on clear liquids until the digestive system resumes normal functioning. The patient will need to at least pass gas before he or she can resume eating, so let the nurse know when it happens. This is one of the few times you'll be happy to hear your loved one pass gas, and you may both get a giggle out of it, too!

A word about room assignments: When Bryan returned from surgery once, he was reassigned to a room in the Telemetry Department, where they could monitor him more closely. I was a little upset about having to change nurses after I had gotten attached to one set. However, I knew it was better for Bryan to be moved to a location with a lower staff-to-patient ratio and the ability to keep a closer eye on him. The nurses there were just as nice and just as caring, and we came to love and appreciate them, too.

Take only what you need.

Another thing that bothered me was moving all the things I had taken to the hospital from one room to another. I had my pre-packed tote bag, but I had a tendency to bring one or two things each day I went back, from crossword puzzle books, to car magazines, to DVDs (when we had a DVD player in the room). That made it much harder to pack everything when Bryan was moved to a new room. I finally learned not to take more than I could carry easily in one trip, and not to leave anything in the room except Bryan's clothes.

The patient's time in the hospital won't be any longer than absolutely necessary. Your doctor and health care provider both want the patient out of the hospital as soon as possible, to keep their costs down. Don't be upset with your doctor when you hear that your loved one needs to stay another day or so. It's for the patient's benefit to stay when the doctor says so. And trust me, it's easier to stay an extra day than go back to the emergency room and get readmitted if your loved one was sent home too soon.

TREATMENT STEP 4—WHEN SURGERY WON'T HELP

One of the first thoughts to cross your mind when you hear that your loved one has cancer is, *Take it out of there—now!* Surgery is the quickest way to remove a tumor, but there are times when surgery is not a viable treatment. In those cases, the oncologist can recommend and possibly perform other procedures.

Chemotherapy

Chemotherapy, the most frequent treatment of choice, is a method of using drugs to shrink or kill the tumors. See "Treatment Step 5—What is chemotherapy? Will it help?" for a description of the process and hints on how to deal with it.

Radiation

Radiation, another form of treatment, is usually coupled with chemotherapy or drug therapy. "Treatment Step 6—What is radiation?" goes into detail on this treatment and what to expect.

If your loved one's doctor says that the cancer is inoperable, don't just lie down and accept it. Ask for a second and possibly a third opinion. Your oncologist won't mind, and will in fact expect it. Check with the health care provider to see if it will pay for the second opinion. Any further opinions will likely not be covered.

In Bryan's case, there was a panel of doctors from multiple specialties who met regularly to discuss diagnoses. Our oncologist had said the tumor was inoperable, but the surgeon on the panel wasn't convinced. He referred Bryan for a PET scan to get a wider picture of the tumors and make the final decision.

Additional Treatment Centers

You may see and hear advertisements for various types of treatment centers with glowing reports of healing. You may want to look into them, but be sure to consider all the components:

- Reliability of the center.
- Cost of travel and hotel stay for multiple visits.
- Cost of doctors and treatment (because your loved one's health care will probably not foot the bill).
- Taking time off work and away from family, etc.

These centers are usually in business to make a profit, so they're not cheap. Ask if they have a scholarship program or some other way of lowering the costs.

You can also check out the American Cancer Society at *www.cancer.org*, the National Cancer Institute at *www.cancer.gov*, and other reputable cancer organizations.

There is ongoing research on new and improved treatment methods, and some organizations may help with expenses if you're willing to take part in experimental procedures.

Be sure to discuss with your oncologist what alternatives you're looking into and trying. Your loved one's treatment will need to be coordinated, and you don't want anything that may interfere with the cure.

No matter what, don't just give up! Life is much too valuable to throw it away. Commit yourselves to the fight, no matter how long it may take. You are both worth it.

TREATMENT STEP 5—WHAT IS CHEMOTHERAPY? WILL IT HELP?

Cancer is basically abnormal cells that grow out of control. Chemotherapy, called "chemo" for short, is a treatment with drugs infused into the body to inhibit the growth and possibly shrink or kill the tumor.

Some cancers respond to chemotherapy in a pill or liquid that can be taken at home. Others respond to a shot administered in a doctor's office. Most chemotherapy involves multiple treatments at a hospital or treatment center.

Chemotherapy involves several treatments.

The drugs are administered in several visits, infused into the bloodstream by way of an intravenous line (IV). Some patients will have an IV inserted every time they have a chemo treatment. Others will have a more permanent tube or port in the chest or abdomen, so they won't be needle-poked at every visit. If nurses have a difficult time drawing your loved one's blood or inserting an IV, the doctor may have a port inserted to protect the veins.

The frequency of the chemo will depend on the type of cancer and the doctor's recommended treatment. Some patients have a treatment five days a week for two to six weeks at a time. Others are scheduled once a week for several weeks. Your loved one's treatment schedule will be customized to his or her cancer and situation. There will likely be time between treatments to give the body a chance to rest, rehydrate, and let the chemicals work.

Your loved one may need to go through several rounds of treatment, such as three weeks on and one week off, for several months. Ask your doctor what this treatment regimen will be, and write it down so you don't forget it.

A chemo treatment is usually done in a room with several chairs, so there will be other people getting their treatments at the same time. Some rooms may have a television or music piped in, but usually not. You may want to take a book, some magazines, or crossword-puzzle books to help pass the time.

The patient's chairs are similar to a dentist's chair, able to recline but not very comfortable. You can ask for a small pillow to put behind your loved one's lower back while sitting. A treatment may take from 30 minutes to several hours. Ask your doctor how long the infusion will be so you can plan accordingly.

If the patient is able to drive to chemotherapy, ask the doctor if the patient will be physically able to drive home after the treatment. If not, have someone else drive. The driver may not need to stay the entire time, but will need to be around to help the patient when the treatment is done.

Fasting or eating before chemotherapy

Your doctor may also recommend that your loved one eat or fast prior to chemo, depending on the type of chemicals he'll be using and whether they're likely to cause nausea. Be sure to follow all his suggestions. He has worked with other patients and knows how to keep side effects at a minimum. Ask if he would recommend that the patient have some snacks while getting treatment. We saw many patients eating lunch while receiving their chemo, so food may help keep nausea away.

Your doctor will run some tests at the end of each round of treatments to see how the cancer is responding. That way, he can alter the drugs for the next round to be most effective. And you and your loved one get to wait and rest until the next treatment.

The best way for a patient to get through a chemo treatment is just to relax and let it run its course. Don't try to hurry it up by increasing the flow in the IV when no one is looking. That may do more harm than good. The doctors and nurses have done this procedure many times before, and they know what's best for this cancer. Let them help you in your fight.

TREATMENT STEP 6—
WHAT IS RADIATION?

Radiation therapy is treatment with high-energy rays or particles, such as x-rays, gamma rays, protons, neutrons, or other sources, to kill cancer cells and shrink tumors. It is also called irradiation, radiotherapy, and x-ray therapy. Radiation is a treatment used in about half of all cancer cases.

When radiation is prescribed following surgery, the tissues affected by the surgery must be given time to heal, usually about a month. Radiation is normally not started until chemotherapy is completed. However, sometimes chemo and radiation are performed together. Your oncologist will prescribe the best therapy for this cancer.

Radiation may be administered externally (from outside the body) or internally (from inside the body), also called brachytherapy.

External Radiation

External radiation is normally done as an outpatient, so your loved one won't be hospitalized for the treatment. Setting up may take some time, but the radiation itself takes only a few minutes. The procedure is painless and much like an x-ray. Careful measurements are taken to determine the exact location, angle, and dose required to hit and treat only the cancer. Anything on the skin, such as lotions, deodorants, antiperspirants, or powders, may interfere with the laser, so be sure your loved one follows the doctor's instructions when preparing for this therapy.

Internal Radiation

For internal radiation, radioactive pellets or seeds in a small container called an implant are placed in the body next to the cancer. The implant may be in the form of thin wires, catheters (plastic tubes), ribbons, or capsules. This treatment may require a hospital stay.

Another form of internal radiation involves radiopharmaceuticals. These are drugs such as radioactive iodine injected into the body, which will leave the body within a few weeks. Take extra caution to follow the doctor's instructions for hand washing, having the patient use different utensils from other family members, and having him or her stay at least an arm's length from anyone who will spend more than two hours in a 24-hour period next to the patient.

External radiation does not make the patient or any part of the body radioactive. However, with internal radiation, the radioactivity remains inside the body, so your loved one will need to stay in the hospital, isolated from hospital staff and visitors for a short time. While the whole body is not radioactive, the area around the implant is, and everyone else must be protected from its effects.

Sometimes external and internal radiations are used simultaneously to increase the intensity and improve the outcome. The procedures are done much the same, but will likely require a short stay in the hospital due to the strength of the radiation.

Many specialists are involved in radiation treatment.

Your loved one will likely have several medical specialists involved in the radiation treatment, in addition to the oncologist:

- Radiation oncologist, who prescribes the treatment.
- Dosimetrist, who determines the proper dose.
- Radiation physicist, who makes sure the machine works properly.
- Radiation therapist, who gives the treatment.

The radiation oncologist will work with the oncologist, surgeon, and all others on the team to coordinate efforts and plan one total course of therapy.

TREATMENT STEP 7—CHEMOTHERAPY WON'T WORK. WHAT NOW?

Cancer treatments continue to improve, giving cancer patients more hope and a longer life expectancy. As of 2009, *more than half* of all people with cancer now live five years or longer after their diagnosis.[2] Effective treatment can prolong and improve your loved one's quality of life.

Most cancer patients survive!

There are numerous other treatments besides the usual chemotherapy, radiation, and surgery. Some are experimental, while others are available today. As research continues, more treatments or therapies may yet be discovered. Your oncologist will very likely be aware of these and will consider them for this cancer fight. This is just for your information.

Anti-Angiogenesis or Angiogenesis Inhibitors Therapy

Anti-angiogenesis or angiogenesis inhibitors therapy affects the formation of new blood cells. Angiogenesis is the body's process of forming new blood vessels, which is controlled by certain chemicals produced in the body. New blood vessels can feed a tumor and help it to grow, so inhibiting the growth of new blood vessels will also inhibit the tumor's growth. This treatment does not affect healthy cells and has only mild side effects. However, anti-angiogenesis can affect the immune system, making the patient more susceptible to infection.

Biological Therapy

Biological therapy can also be called immunotherapy, biotherapy, or biological response modifier therapy. This uses the body's immune system to fight

---

[2] *http://www.cancer.org/Treatment/TreatmentsandSideEffects/TreatmentTypes/ Anti-angiogenesisTreatment/anti-angiogenesis-treatment-defining*

cancer or lessen side effects. Antibodies, which are normally produced in the body and now reproduced in the laboratory, attack foreign substances in the body. This is what helps you fight off a cold or the flu. Advances have allowed doctors to create antibodies that will fight cancer cells as well.

Bone Marrow Transplant

Bone marrow transplant, or **peripheral blood stem cell transplant**, is used to replace bone marrow damaged by disease or cancer treatment such as chemotherapy and radiation. Everyone's body needs good bone marrow to produce blood cells. Bone marrow has been successfully transplanted since 1968. Twenty years later, cells from circulating blood (peripheral blood stem cells) were first used for successful transplant. Stem cells can be donated by the patient, the patient's twin, a family member, or another person whose blood stem cells match the patient's closely. The possibility of transplant allows the oncologist to use stronger doses of chemotherapy or radiation, since the transplant will help your loved one's body to repair itself.

Gene Therapy

Gene therapy is an experimental treatment that involves inserting genetic material into a person's cells to fight the cancer. DNA or RNA may be instilled to repair a cell's damage or to give it a new function. A gene may also be introduced into a cell that will make that cell able to recognize and attack cancer cells. This is most useful in treating inherited diseases and may be used to prevent those diseases. One day, gene therapy may be widely available and effective in treating cancer.

Hyperthermia

Hyperthermia, also called thermal therapy or thermotherapy, is a method of exposing body tissue to temperatures up to 113° F, which affects cancer cells with little damage to normal cells. It is usually done along with radiation and/or chemotherapy and causes those treatments to be more effective. Hyperthermia can be performed internally for tumors deep inside the body, externally for tumors on or near the skin, or endocavitary for tumors in or near body cavities. It can be localized to one area of the body or performed on the entire body if the cancer has metastasized or spread.

Laser Therapy

Laser therapy is light that is focused into a very narrow beam that can perform delicate surgery, such as tumor removal with minimal cutting, bleeding, and risk of infection. It is used mostly on tumors on the skin's surface or on the lining of internal organs. The heat of the laser seals off blood vessels, reduces bleeding, and keeps the area sterile. Laser therapy may be performed on an out-patient basis with no hospital stay.

Photodynamic Therapy

Photodynamic therapy, or PDT, uses drugs that are activated by certain kinds of light and has been used to treat cancer for more than 100 years. The drugs are injected into the body and absorbed mainly by cancer cells. One to three days later, the cancerous area is exposed to light, activating the drugs. It is used mainly on the surface or just under the surface of the skin, places that light can reach. The light can pass through tissue up to one centimeter thick. PDT may work as well as a combination of surgery and radiation for certain cancers, with fewer side effects and little or no scarring. However, it can only be used when the cancer has not spread.

Targeted Cancer Therapy

Targeted cancer therapy is a new treatment using drugs or enzymes to cause the cancer cells to die or at least to stop growing, giving chemotherapy a better chance of shrinking the tumor. Targeted therapy doesn't damage blood cells or bone marrow like some other treatments, and is usually used in coordination with other treatments like chemotherapy and radiation. This is a relatively new method of treatment, and there are multiple drugs that can target just the cancer cells with little damage to normal cells.

Vaccines

Vaccines, normally used to prevent a disease, can be used to treat an existing cancer, to stop its growth, or to kill any cancer cells not eliminated by other treatment. It boosts the body's immune system to fight foreign objects, including cancer cells. Some cancers can be prevented by administering the vaccine to a healthy person. Other vaccines are being developed to stop cancer growth, shrink tumors, and kill cancer cells not eliminated by other treatments.

This is *not* a checklist to discuss with your doctor. Many of these therapies are limited as to the type of cancer they can treat, so don't assume that your oncologist will try every method of treatment available. Your doctor is well-informed on all these treatments as well as experimental therapies and will only use those that have a good chance of shrinking or killing this particular type of cancer.

TREATMENT STEP 8—SHOULD WE TRY ALTERNATIVE FORMS OF MEDICINE?

By all means, try anything within reason that may help. Be sure to discuss with your doctor any alternatives your loved one considers trying, and let him or her know when you do try one. You want these attempts to work with, not against, what your doctor is doing. Together, you can be more effective in this fight.

Doctors and researchers have yet to discover the cause of cancer, and a definitive cure continues to elude them. Western medicine has traditional cures that may work against some cancers, but not all. It only makes sense that you would want to try every possible chance of getting rid of this cancer.

There are alternatives.

Some alternative forms of medicine are:

- Exercise.
- Healthy eating.
- Homeopathy.
- Acupuncture.

Exercise

Exercise can encourage everyone's body to work at optimum levels. WebMD reports that "exercise and eating right can help prevent people from getting cancer. The latest information shows that exercise for cancer patients can also keep cancer from recurring."[3] On that same website, Kerry Courneya, PhD, professor and Canada Research Chair in Physical Activity and Cancer at the University of Alberta in Edmonton, Canada, states, "Several recent studies suggest that higher levels of physical activity are associated with a

---

[3] http://www.webmd.com/cancer/features/exercise-cancer-patients

reduced risk of the cancer coming back, and a longer survival after a cancer diagnosis."[4]

Remain as physically active as possible.

The American Cancer Society reports, "It is important for a person with cancer to remain as physically active as possible. Exercise as much as your condition allows to help keep muscles functioning as well as possible."[5] This website also states that exercise programs benefit cancer patients' recovery.

Not only does exercise get you in physical shape, but it can improve the patient's mental outlook. In other words, the patient will feel better. Check with your loved one's doctor, and encourage him or her to do as much exercise as possible to keep mobile and in the best shape possible. Bryan stopped moving and just lay on the couch, causing loss of muscle tone. He eventually had trouble keeping his balance, even with a walker. Exercise might have helped him, but we didn't know it at the time.

Healthy Eating

According to the National Cancer Institute at their website *www.cancer.gov*, people with cancer have different dietary needs. For most people, a healthy diet consists of fruits and vegetables, modest amounts of meat and milk products, and small amounts of fat, sugar, alcohol, and salt. However, when someone has cancer, he or she needs to keep up strength to deal with the side effects of treatment. As Bryan's Hospice doctor told us, the cancer is screaming at your brain to not eat, so just eating can be an overwhelming challenge.

Your loved one may need extra protein and calories, possibly extra milk, cheese, eggs, or food supplements such as Ensure. If they have trouble chewing or swallowing, you could add sauces and gravies. You can also find a protein powder at your grocery or health-food store to add to soups, milkshakes, cooked cereal, or just about any other mixed food. One warning: too much protein powder can affect the flavor or texture of food, so use it in moderation.

---

[4] Ibid.

[5] *http://www.cancer.org/docroot/MIT/MIT_2_1x_ExerciseToStayActive.asp*

Homeopathy (also spelled Homoeopathy)

Homeopathy (pronounced ho-me-OP-a-thy), also known as homeopathic medicine, is a system using natural, concentrated medicines. Developed in Germany more than 200 years ago, it has been used in the United States since the early 1900s. Homeopathy can be used for wellness and prevention in addition to the treatment of diseases, conditions, and side effects.

A homeopath (homeopathy doctor) treats patients based on their personal health history, body type, genetics, and current status, including physical, mental, and emotional symptoms. Treatments are custom-tailored to each patient. It is not unusual for two people with the same disease or condition to receive different treatments.

Homeopathic remedies include natural substances from animals, minerals, or plants such as red onions and stinging nettle plant. The quality of homeopathic products is governed by the Federal Food, Drug, and Cosmetic Act of 1938 and is regulated the same as nonprescription, over-the-counter medications. These remedies are prepared following guidelines of the "Homeopathic Pharmacopoeia of the United States" (HPUS).

My friend Allison Groves tells of her husband, Dave's, fight using homeopathy. After getting Dave released from the hospital, Allison took him to her homeopathist, who put him on a regimen of vitamins, herbs, and minerals. Within two months, Dave was cancer-free. His oncologist performed two PET scans to confirm this. Unfortunately, Dave didn't want to take pills for the rest of his life. He stopped the homeopathic remedies, and his cancer returned.

If you find that homeopathy works to rid your loved one's body of the cancer, by all means encourage him or her continue to use it. If pills will save his or her life, please have your loved one take the pills!

Acupuncture

Acupuncture is a procedure of stimulating one's nerves by inserting and manipulating fine needles into specific points on the body to relieve pain or for therapeutic purposes. This form of treatment, discovered centuries ago in China, holds that by stimulating nerve endings, the body could be encouraged to heal itself. Some people consider it "woo-woo" medicine, but Bryan and I had used it successfully for ruptured spinal disks, carpal tunnel, and grief in dealing with personal problems.

Acupuncture may not be able to cure cancer, but it can be very effective in the treatment of pain and side effects associated with cancer and its treatment. An acupuncture treatment takes less than one hour. It involves lying comfortably on an exam table with your torso covered. For my last acupuncture treatment, I just rolled up my sleeves to the shoulders and pant legs to the knees. Then, the doctor inserts needles thinner than a strand of hair, which doesn't even hurt. If the needles do hurt, the acupuncturist is doing it wrong.

Once the needles are in place, you get to lie there and nap for 30 minutes. It's hard to believe that you can sleep with needles in your body, but it's surprisingly relaxing. The needles do their thing while you just rest. When you finally wake up, you are so calm, it's hard to stay awake to drive home. Be sure your loved one has a driver until you know how the acupuncture will affect him or her.

Acupuncture may cure or ease pain.

In some cases, acupuncture can help to cure a disease or disorder. In others, it helps to deal with pain or emotional problems. Appointments may be once or twice a week to begin with, but after a while the treatments may be less frequent for maintenance.

Whatever form of treatment you and your loved one choose, give it your all until you feel it is no longer working. It's just like being on a diet: Whatever you do to lose weight is what you'll need to do to keep the weight off. Whatever method your loved one chooses to treat cancer must be followed through to its completion. If stopped too soon, the treatment may be ineffective.

One exception is that if one treatment is not working or is doing more harm than good, stop it and try another form of action. Don't jeopardize your loved one's health by being stubborn. Be sure to discuss all treatment options with your oncologist.

TREATMENT STEP 9—
HOSPICE PALLIATIVE CARE

"My doctor just referred me to hospice for palliative care. Does that mean he's given up on me and I'm going to die?" That's the first question that comes to mind when your oncologist says that your loved one has been referred to hospice. That's what my husband Bryan and my friend Mark thought. Both of them asked me the same question just a few months apart.

The word *hospice* has an ominous sound to it. Most people see it as the final step. But stop and think: *hospice* comes from the same root word as *hospitality*, which is the act of providing care, comfort, and kindness where it is needed. That's what hospice does: it provides care, comfort and kindness where and when it is needed the most.

Palliative care provides comfort during treatment.

There are two hospice services. The first is palliative care, which is just to provide comfort while the patient undergoes treatment. The second is hospice, which is when treatment has stopped and all that is done for the patient is comfort.

While your oncologist is busy treating and fighting your loved one's cancer, you and the patient may need a little extra attention and help in dealing with day-to-day living. Your loved one may need pain management, prescriptions delivered as soon as possible, a medical expert on call 24 hours a day, and a nurse and doctor who make house calls, to save you frequent trips to the doctor's office and keep symptoms and side effects under control.

That's what hospice does. They take over managing the patient's personal comfort, freeing your oncologist to focus on treatment. Your oncologist has not given up. He's just called for some reinforcements in the fight.

When Bryan was nauseated or needed help to sleep, all we had to do was call our hospice nurse and explain the problem. Then, the appropriate medical supply or prescription was delivered to our front door within a few hours. With that kind of help, I didn't have to load him into the car, sit in the doctor's office for an appointment, and wait while a prescription was filled. It conserved his energy (and mine) and brought comfort to our home when we really needed it.

Before my friend Mark Cerdena was referred to hospice, he had to drive himself to the pharmacy every time he needed a prescription. He was tired from his treatments, but had no other option, as his wife had to keep working. Having hospice deliver his meds saved his energy and allowed him to rest.

Hospice also gave us the added benefit of a twice-weekly visit from a nurse's aide. The aide can help the patient bathe or shower, give neck massages, change bed linens, or sit with the patient while the caregiver goes out for an hour. That's when I got my grocery shopping done, since I couldn't leave Bryan alone.

Another plus was that all hospice expenses were covered by Medicare. That meant that all those co-pays, prescription charges, and other costs weren't continually chipping away at our checking account. Anything that Bryan needed was brought to our door, from pills to wound dressing to a bed wedge. They even offered a bedside toilet (which Bryan refused to use) and a hospital bed (which he also refused). It was such a relief to not have to go out and buy or rent all those things. Check with your medical insurance carrier or hospice to see if their charges will be covered.

Hospice is another word for *help*, and it comes at a time when you really need all the help you can get. We were very thankful that our doctor called in the troops to help us fight the daily discomforts that took such a huge toll on Bryan. They helped me as Bryan's caregiver, too.

TREATMENT STEP 10—
WHAT IS HOSPICE, REALLY?

Hospice is a program of care for people who are near the end of their lives, allowing them to live an alert, pain-free life at home, in a hospital, in a nursing home, or in a hospice facility.

Hospice affirms life.

The philosophy of hospice accepts death as the final stage of life and neither postpones nor hastens death. It affirms life and the necessity of providing a quality and dignity of life for patients and their loved ones. Hospice provides medical, psychological, and spiritual help to terminally ill patients and their families by professionals and volunteers dedicated to your loved one's comfort.

Too often, hospice is not started soon enough, and the patient lives with far more pain than is necessary. Then, by the time a referral to hospice is made, it's difficult to lower the pain to a manageable level.

Palliative care from hospice provides comfort to a cancer patient while the oncologist continues treatment. At this stage, palliative care takes over the management of the patient's pain, physical issues, and side effects.

Hospice treats the patient rather than the disease, and is intended for a time when cancer is no longer treated and the patient has six months or fewer to live. It provides comfort and freedom from pain, so the patient can enjoy his or her family as long as possible.

A patient, doctor, or family member may feel that calling in hospice means that there is no hope and that everyone is giving up. This isn't necessarily true. If cancer goes into remission, your loved one can be taken out of the hospice program and receive active cancer treatment.

When Bryan was first admitted to hospice, their doctor was concerned about the number of prescriptions he was taking. After Bryan became anemic and was sleeping all the time, the doctor sat down with us, reviewed our list of 19 medications, and narrowed it down to a more manageable amount that didn't drug him as much. He was then more alert with minimal pain, which helped both of us.

Family members are main caregivers during in-home hospice care.

Most hospice care is provided in the home, with family members serving as the main caregivers. Family members are included in decisions about the patient's care. Often, patients can't think as clearly as before and can't make decisions on their own, so it helps to have at least one family member discuss the decisions and carry out the instructions.

In-home hospice care is provided by a nurse or a doctor who actually makes house calls, believe it or not! They are also available by phone 24 hours a day, 7 days a week. At times, I had to call late at night for help, and a nurse came to our house within an hour. Other times, they can assist over the phone, offering advice and having prescriptions or medical supplies delivered as soon as they are needed.

Hospice provides respite for caregivers by having a nurse's aide visit twice a week. No matter how much you love the person fighting cancer, you can't be around 24 hours a day and always be at your best. You need some time away to recharge, if only to go out to the driveway and sit in your car for an hour. I used that time to do grocery shopping, go to the bank, or just cry. Our aide James would change the sheets, shave Bryan, or just sit while Bryan slept.

Hospice provides a chaplain and a counselor who make personal visits and phone calls to help the patient and the caregiver with whatever they need. This is a time when you need all the spiritual and emotional help you can get, and they're more than willing to help you.

Hospice allows your loved one to live and die comfortably and with dignity. They are God's hands with skin on, touching us when we need it most.

PHYSICAL STEPS

PHYSICAL STEP 1—POSSIBLE SIDE EFFECTS OF TREATMENT

Cancer and its treatment may produce uncomfortable side effects. Not everyone will suffer from these, but anticipating and being prepared are the best ways to handle them.

Among possible side effects are pain, nausea and vomiting, loose stools, bleeding and bruising, anemia, fatigue, hair loss, and infection. The patient may get one or more of these, so knowing how to control them will help in your loved one's journey.

It's much harder to reduce pain than to control it.

Pain

Pain is often an indicator of cancer, so most patients have already dealt with it. When in a hospital, the nurses will ask the patient to give their pain a number from 0 (no pain) to 10 (the worst pain ever). It's best if the patient can be honest with him or herself about the pain level. If it goes above 3, the patient can take something to ease the pain. It's much harder to reduce pain than to control it.

When Bryan was in pain, he would wait until the level reached 8 before he asked for help, and then had to wait an hour or longer for the meds to take effect and ease the pain. When we finally convinced him to take a small dose of pain meds every few hours to keep the pain low, he could function more normally.

Nausea, Vomiting, or Loose Stools

Stomach upset cannot be ignored, but it can be controlled. It affects not only the patient's ability to eat and fight the cancer, but also the desire to carry on a normal life.

Here are some ways to reduce stomach upset. Have the patient:

- Drink water throughout the day to stay hydrated.
- Eat and drink slowly.
- Eat 5-6 small meals a day instead of 3 normal-sized meals.
- Eat bland foods that are easy on the stomach.
- Sit up or go for a walk after eating.
- Stay away from foods that are too hot or too cold.

Eating ginger is a natural way of coping with stomach upset. Your grocer will have a variety of products containing ginger. You might try tea, ginger cookies, or crystallized ginger candy. Ask your doctor about over-the-counter medications before you try them. You don't want to aggravate the situation or counteract ongoing treatment.

Bleeding or Bruising

See "Physical Step 3—Bleeding" for details, but here are a few ideas to help you cope:

- Be careful with anything sharp that might cut your loved one's skin.
- Call your doctor the first time you see blood or unexpected bruising.
- If bleeding from the mouth, sucking on ice chips may slow or stop the bleeding. (This is a good hint with children. A frozen Popsicle works well, too.) If your loved one's mouth is still bleeding after 30 minutes, call the doctor.
- Give the patient a soft toothbrush to reduce gum bleeding.
- When there is more than one cup of blood with a bowel movement, call your doctor.
- Have the patient wear shoes or slippers at all times.

Anemia

Anemia is a condition when one's body doesn't have enough red blood cells, which can make the patient feel very weak or tired. This cannot be treated at home, so call your doctor if you detect any of these symptoms in your loved one:

- Feels dizzy or faint.
- Experiences shortness of breath.
- Feels more tired or weaker than normal.
- Heart starts beating very fast.
- Has chest pain.
- Hands or feet swell.
- Skin becomes very pale.

Treating anemia may involve eating foods rich in nutrients, taking iron or folic acid supplements, and stopping any bleeding. Your doctor will determine the best treatment, but it's up to you and your loved one to follow his advice.

We were unaware of the possibility of anemia until Bryan fell one night, and even his walker couldn't keep him upright. He cut his ear on a piece of furniture and ended up with 20 stitches and a gauze turban for a week.

Fatigue

Your loved one may find him or herself feeling more tired than normal. Don't let them try to do everything alone. Have them do only what they absolutely must do. Take time off from work, work fewer hours, or work at home if at all possible to help. Let others do things for you. Learn to ask for help.

Be sure to have your loved one eat healthy foods and drink liquids all day to keep his or her body working and fighting. Have your loved one drink water in sips instead of gulps and exercise if at all possible, even if only 15 minutes a day, to keep his or her energy level up.

When your loved one needs a rest, have him or her lie down. Help him or her learn to power nap. Bryan took short naps almost every day of his adult life, so that was an easy thing to continue during his cancer journey. Those 20 minutes can give your loved one a much-needed energy boost in the middle of the day.

Power naps can help your loved one get much-needed energy.

Hair Loss

Some cancer treatments can cause hair to fall out in as little as two to three weeks. It may come out in clumps while shampooing or brushing, or just on the pillow. Hair loss is often temporary, as the hair can start to grow back even before therapy is completed. You may lose hair—not only from your head but from any place on your body.

Hair loss can be minimized by being gentle when washing or brushing the hair and wearing a hair net at night. Also, avoid hair styles that pull on the hair, such as pony tails or braids. You may want to minimize the effect of hair falling out by cutting the hair short or shaving the head when you first notice hair loss.

If your loved one wants a wig, buy it before treatment or as soon as you can, while he or she still feels like shopping. Your doctor can write a prescription for the wig so that health insurance will cover it. Consider buying two wigs, one for everyday use and one for special occasions. One friend didn't think to buy a wig before her treatment started, and she was too weak to go shopping after her hair loss. Unfortunately, wigs that were brought to her house didn't fit, and she ended up just wearing scarves.

Instead of a wig, your loved one may prefer a scarf or a turban. Choose cotton, which will stay on a smooth scalp better than nylon, silk, or polyester. And don't forget sunscreen for a bare scalp.

When the hair starts to grow, it will require gentle treatment at first, so wait a few months for perms or hair coloring, which may cause it to break. Keeping a short hairdo will help hair to regain its strength.

Infection

Call your doctor if your loved one's symptoms include:

- Chills.
- A temperature of 100.5° F or higher.
- Ear pain.
- Cough or sore throat.
- Bloody or cloudy urine.
- A rash.
- Sores in the mouth or on the tongue.
- Swelling or redness, especially with a port or catheter.

These are symptoms of infection that should be controlled as soon as possible. A cancer patient's body cannot fight infection normally, so you'll need all the help you can get.

PHYSICAL STEP 2—NAUSEA

Your loved one may have nausea with chemotherapy or radiation, or even before treatments start. Cancer is notorious for not only taking away the desire for food but also upsetting the stomach. The patient may be nauseated with or without vomiting. Be sure your loved one drinks enough liquids so he or she doesn't become dehydrated if vomiting. The patient may end up in the emergency room to have IV fluids pumped in.

Tell your doctor or nurse if your loved one feels nauseated or is vomiting. There are medicines that can control both, some over-the-counter and some only available by prescription. Taking these on a regular basis to keep the nausea under control is easier than trying to get rid of it once you're miserable.

Another thing that may help is eating 6-8 small meals a day instead of three large meals. The stomach won't have time to completely empty out and become upset. That's why cruise lines will offer food all day long—if there's food in your stomach, you're less likely to get nauseated. It works on dry land, too.

Serve six to eight small meals instead of three large meals a day.

Some foods have the ability to settle your stomach. Among these are crackers, dry cereals, toast, non-greasy foods, bland (not spicy) foods like Cream of Wheat or chicken soup, gelatin, Popsicles, ginger, hard candies, and warm or cool drinks, not hot or ice cold.

You may have these on hand or can readily find them at your local grocer. Several of our friends recommended ginger, so I shopped for every product with ginger in it. At our grocery store, I found ginger tea (some with honey-lemon), ginger cookies (three different types), ginger ale (it may help to let the fizz out of it), ground ginger in the spice aisle to add to just about anything, fresh ginger in the produce section, and crystallized ginger in the candy aisle.

There are also some foods that may add to nausea, which you would be wise to avoid. Among these are spicy foods, fried foods, rich foods, some spices, and fatty foods, including ice cream. Use your own judgment. If it gave your loved one heartburn before, it will again. Even so, there may be some foods that your loved one could eat before that present a problem now. Just remember to write it down so you don't repeat the mistake.

A good rule to follow is to stay away from favorite foods when nauseated. That much-loved pizza or ice cream may upset your loved one's stomach, and he or she will never be able to eat it again. Your loved one doesn't want to have to give up favorite foods along with everything else that's already been given up.

The body is working to fight cancer, so eat light.

Also, don't have the patient eat as much as usual. The body is working hard to fight the cancer, and forcing it to digest a stomach full of food may be asking too much.

Your doctor can recommend foods to eat before and after chemotherapy treatments that will calm the stomach. He has seen many patients before, and his knowledge is from past experience. Tell him what works so he can pass that info on to other patients.

PHYSICAL STEP 3—BLEEDING

Seeing one's blood is always a little unnerving, especially when dealing with cancer.

When To Call The Doctor About Bleeding

Call the doctor when your loved one:

- Bleeds for the first time.
- Has significant bleeding from the mouth.
- Has mouth bleeding for 30 minutes that you can't stop.
- Vomits blood that looks like coffee grounds.
- Feels light-headed or dizzy or if they faint.
- Has more than a cup of blood with a bowel movement.
- Has unexpected bruises appear.
- Passes pink urine.

If there is blood in your loved one's mouth after brushing teeth, he or she may have a low platelet count as a result of chemotherapy. Sucking ice chips, rinsing the mouth with ice water, and using a soft toothbrush or foam mouth swabs to brush teeth may help.

When there is an incision, such as for a port or a catheter, the cut will not heal as long as the port is in place. This increases the opportunity for bleeding and possible infection if the incision is not cared for properly. Be sure to follow your doctor's advice for managing the port and reducing the chance of complications.

Preventing Bleeding

To prevent unnecessary bleeding, have your loved one:

- Use an electric shaver, not a razor, to avoid nicks.
- Always wear shoes or slippers.

- Be careful when using scissors, knives, nail clippers, or any other sharp objects.
- Use an extra-soft toothbrush.
- Blow the nose gently.
- Avoid using dental floss or toothpicks.
- Avoid playing rough sports.
- Avoid taking aspirin unless your doctor advises it.
- Use a saline nasal spray.
- Make sure the patient's dentist knows if he or she is undergoing chemotherapy. He or she may need to check a platelet count prior to all dental work.
- Avoid glucosamine with chondroitin or vitamin E, both of which can thin the blood.
- Not take antibiotics when on Coumadin, as this can thin the blood.

Talk with your doctor about any unusual bleeding. Don't take any unnecessary chances. Your loved one is worth it, and bleeding is something that you may be able to control together.

PHYSICAL STEP 4—CAN'T SLEEP

Many cancer patients lie awake at night wondering, imagining, worrying, thinking, planning, and whatever else happens to cross their minds. It's normal, but it doesn't need to be a regular occurrence.

Even before Bryan was diagnosed, he needed help sleeping once in a while. After he heard the "C" word, his mind went to work even harder when the lights went out. He called it "brain noise," that time when your brain goes into overdrive when it's supposed to be in sleep mode.

Follow a routine schedule for sleep.

One of the simplest ways get to sleep is to follow the same schedule every night, even on weekends. This is true whether or not you have cancer. This advice is for both the patient and the caregiver.

Go to bed and get up at the same time every day, so your body gets used to it. You'll be surprised to find yourself eventually waking at the same time every day, even without an alarm clock.

Give yourself 30 to 60 minutes of late-night downtime to help your body slow down in preparation for a good night's sleep. This time can be spent reading a book, watching television, petting the dog or cat, or just talking.

Avoid watching the news.

I learned that watching the local news programs right before bed would affect the quality of my sleep. After hearing all the terrible things that happened in my town and around the world, I would have trouble falling asleep or have wild, unsettling dreams several nights a week. Bryan finally learned the same lesson, and we started watching news in the morning instead.

After your downtime, go through the same routine every night to get ready for bed. Change your clothes, brush your teeth, and do whatever you need to do each night, always in the same order. If you follow the same process regularly, your brain will learn that sleep is the final step, and you'll find yourself drifting off sooner.

Where you sleep and sleep position can have a direct effect on the quality of rest you get. Although Bryan slept on a waterbed for decades, that mattress was no longer comfortable after cancer. He could sleep on the innerspring mattress in the guest room, so we replaced our waterbed mattress with an innerspring mattress and a memory foam pad. This alleviated the pressure on his joints resting on the mattress, allowing him to wake up with fewer aches and pains.

A bed wedge can facilitate sleep.

A bed wedge can help you get more restful sleep as well. Even though Bryan had always slept on his side, he could now sleep better on his back with his head elevated. He used two pillows at first to raise his head. Later, he used a bed wedge, which was larger and stayed in place better than piling up the pillows. This kept him from becoming congested and allowed his breathing to be more regular, resulting in better sleep.

Warmth is necessary for good sleep. Have you ever tried to sleep when you're cold, maybe on a camping trip? It doesn't work very well, and when you're ill or have lost weight, it's harder to maintain body heat. Not only did Bryan use an extra blanket, but he also wore socks and slippers all day every day and had the thermostat set a few degrees higher than normal. Being a little warm was a minor sacrifice on my part so that Bryan could be comfortable and get more rest.

You may request sleep aids from your doctor.

Natural, non-medical products can help you get to sleep. A cup of decaffeinated tea can be very calming, especially with quiet conversation. Many tea companies have blends specifically for sleep, such as chamomile teas or Sleepytime by Celestial Seasonings. Don't make the mistake of having chocolate chip cookies or a piece of chocolate cake along with the tea. The caffeine in the sweets may keep you awake.

If your loved one needs a sleeping pill, an over-the-counter sleep aid may work, but check with your doctor first. You don't want him or her to take anything that may interfere with other medications being taken or any treatment being received. You can start with half a pill, increasing if more is needed, but only with doctor's approval.

As a caregiver, you probably won't want to take a sleep aid. If your loved one needs you in the middle of the night, you may find it hard to wake up to help.

There may be times when your loved one needs even more help to get to sleep. Your doctor can prescribe various sleep aids. Be aware of how they affect the patient. The patient may sleep for hours on end, or can take the pills in moderation so he or she is awake when he or she wants to be, and asleep when he or she prefers. If one medication doesn't work, let your doctor know and you can try another.

Keep at it until you find the best process or medication for a sleep routine for both you and your loved one. Your bodies need rest, so do whatever it takes to get that rest. You can train your brain to learn when it's supposed to shut off, and you can make you bed comfortable. You may still have an occasional bout with insomnia, but it shouldn't be as often.

PHYSICAL STEP 5—SLEEPING ALL THE TIME

Having any type of serious illness or being a caregiver can drain what little energy you have, resulting in excessive sleeping. In other words, sickness or caregiving can make you tired, which in turn makes you sleep, maybe more than you want to.

Sometimes it's better to sleep, like at night or when you want the time to pass more quickly. If you and your loved one have no trouble sleeping at night, be thankful. There are many folks who have trouble falling asleep or staying asleep who would love to be in your shoes. It's the daytime sleeping that can present problems.

Pain meds can cause sleepiness.

Pain medications can have drowsiness as a side effect. They tend to dull the nervous system, which in turn dulls the brain and makes the patient want to sleep. But taking something to ease the pain doesn't need to knock the patient out.

As I explained earlier, Bryan tried to "be a man" and withstand the pain, letting it reach 8 on a scale from 0 to 10 before he'd ask for help. We convinced him to take a low dose of pain meds every few hours to keep the pain lower. This prevented him from taking a large dosage to lower the pain level, which made him sleep for several hours.

Whether you're the patient or the caregiver, you probably don't want to sleep all the time. You may still need to function, keep working, or drive a car, so be sure to talk with your doctor. You don't want to jeopardize your job, your safety, or the safety of those around you.

Some drugs will put you to sleep, while others can increase your alertness and give you more energy. You and your doctor can work together to find the best combination for you or your loved one. Something as simple as drinking a cup of coffee or a glass of cola with caffeine may be all you need to keep you awake in order to function normally or receive visitors. Again, talk with your doctor, even about caffeine intake.

PHYSICAL STEP 6—WHAT CAN WE DO ABOUT THE PAIN?

Just because your loved one has cancer doesn't mean that he or she will be in pain. Some cancer patients have no pain at all. However, many do suffer and since most people would rather not feel any pain at all, keeping pain under control will be a priority. The American Cancer Society says that managing pain is part of cancer treatment.[6]

Keep the pain level below 3.

First of all, keep track of your loved one's pain level often each day. Most hospitals will give you a chart to number pain from 0 to 10, with 0 meaning no pain at all and 10 meaning the worst possible pain. They don't want you to let your loved one's pain go above 3, so be sure to (while in the hospital) let the nurse or doctor know if it reaches 4 or higher.

If possible, don't allow the patient to "be tough" like my husband. Bryan would let the pain get up to an 8, and then ask for pain meds. The main problem with letting the pain increase is that it takes a long time and more meds to deal with a pain level of 8 than if meds are taken at a level 4, not to mention the pain itself and the exhaustion it causes. Suffering doesn't make the situation any better and doesn't help in the fight.

We found that giving Bryan a low dose of pain meds every few hours all day kept his pain at bay, and he was much more functional than when he let the pain increase. His doctor was very pleased that we had figured that out, as he didn't have to prescribe multiple pain meds for different levels of pain. Your loved one will likely have one medication for normal pain, and a second for "breakthrough" pain, those times when there is a spike in the pain level.

Keep track of what meds your doctor prescribes, and be sure to give him the list when he prescribes a new medication. You don't want your loved

---

[6] *http://www.cancer.org/acs/groups/cid/documents/webcontent/002906-pdf.pdf*

one to become overly medicated like Bryan, who ended up iron-deficient, passed out, and fell onto a piece of furniture, requiring 20 stitches in his ear.

Follow dosage instructions to the letter.

Follow the instructions with all medications, no matter how you might want to alter them. The meds may work against one another, not work at all, or cause harmful side effects, and you'll be worse off, maybe even find yourselves in the emergency room. If you feel the need to double up the patient's meds or increase the dosage, check with your doctor first. You may want to ask at the time the medication is prescribed how and when you can safely increase the dose, so you know what leeway you have.

Don't worry about your loved one becoming addicted to the pain meds when following the doctor's instructions. Don't let friends or family members talk your loved one out of taking pain meds because of possible addiction. They're not the ones suffering. If the patient hasn't abused drugs in the past, it's unlikely he or she will start now. Also, if taking a drug that includes an opioid (a narcotic like morphine or codeine), the doctor can help to wean the patient off it when it is no longer needed.

If any medication gives a side effect such as nausea, vomiting, itching, constipation, or drowsiness, let your doctor or nurse know. There are other meds available, so you don't need to suffer. Your medical team can work with you to find medication that the body will tolerate better.

Let the doctor know if pain meds don't work.

Be sure to tell your doctor or nurse if the pain doesn't subside after taking a pain med. Some will work better than others, so you may get a different prescription. Also let them know if you need help paying for the drugs.

It helps if your loved one can be specific about where the pain is located, when it came on, what makes it better or worse, what type of pain it is, and anything else about it. Write it down as he or she tells you, so you can relay the information as needed.

Help your loved one identify specific location and level of pain.

Your doctor or nurse needs to know what type of pain it is: sharp, aching, dull, burning, shooting, or whatever. Bryan's favorite phrase was, "I'm half sick," which didn't reveal anything, and didn't help in figuring out how to make it better. When he said instead that he had a stabbing pain in his lower left abdomen, they could do something to help him.

Some pain will respond to other treatments, such as heat, cold, massage, relaxation exercises, or over-the-counter drugs such as ibuprofen, acetaminophen, and aspirin. Check with your doctor to see if these can be taken.

Remember, your loved one's pain management is in your own hands. Your loved one doesn't have to hurt. Just help him or her take control.

PHYSICAL STEP 7—THE PAIN IS GETTING WORSE

God gave us pain to tell us that something is wrong. Pain can be a warning sign of the side effects of treatment or other problems. It's up to you and your loved one to take the steps necessary to get the problem fixed.

Pain can affect the patient's entire life, especially when it keeps getting worse. Your loved one dreads the pain and how it can limit, isolate, and incapacitate him or her. It can affect the ability to eat or sleep. He or she becomes irritable around those who are helping the most. Others don't understand what the patient is feeling and that all the patient wants right now is freedom from the pain.

Having cancer doesn't mean your loved one must be in pain. Controlling cancer pain is a part of the treatment. When pain is controlled, your loved one can eat, sleep, feel, and function better, even enjoy life again. There's no reason not to control the pain.

The first step in pain management is to tell the doctor or nurse. They can't do anything if they don't know what the problem is. There's no reason to "tough it out" and live in agony when help is nearby.

Keep pain from starting and prepare for "breakthrough" pain.

There are numerous methods and medications that can lessen the pain:

- Keep pain from starting, and it'll be much easier to control. Nurses routinely ask patients to rate their pain on a scale of 0, meaning no pain, to 10, meaning the worst possible pain. Don't let your loved one's pain get above 3 without doing something to ease it. It will take a higher dosage of pain meds to get an 8 down to a 3, and there may be side effects.
- Keep a record of the pain level and how it responds to pain medications. This will help the health care team to decide what works best and what dosage. I would ask Bryan to rate

his pain whenever he asked for a pain med, and then rate it again 30 minutes and 60 minutes later. That way, we knew what drugs worked faster and what dosages to use.

- A patient can have "breakthrough" pain when the pain occurs suddenly or for a short time. That's when the patient needs to take something else to bring it down to a 3 again. Ask about a liquid form of the pain med, which may be absorbed into the system faster than a pill. If your loved one has an IV or a port, you may be able to inject a liquid pain med, which will act faster.

- A body does not become immune to pain medications, so don't save the "big guns" for when the pain gets worse. If an over-the-counter pain med doesn't do the trick, try something stronger. Your loved one's body needs it, so give it what it needs.

- Try different combinations of prescription drugs and over-the-counter medications. Bryan was taking a prescription pain pill every six hours, but used liquid ibuprofen for breakthrough pain. The combination didn't make him sleep like a higher dosage of his pain med would, and he was alert when he wanted to be.

- Talk with your doctor about all possibilities. When one method doesn't work, try another and another until you find the best one.

- If you and your doctor can't manage the pain, ask to speak to a pain specialist. This may be an oncologist, an anesthetist, a neurologist, or someone in palliative care. They are experts at various methods and medications to use for a patient's comfort.

Don't worry about your loved one becoming addicted to pain medications. As long as you follow your doctor's dosing instructions and administer pain meds only to manage the pain, there is a very small chance of addiction. As the pain lessens, your doctor can decrease the dosage and wean the patient off medications with no residual craving.

Do whatever is needed to keep your loved one comfortable. He or she has enough to deal with now without being limited by uncontrolled pain.

WAITING STEPS

WAITING STEP 1—WHAT DO WE DO WHILE WAITING FOR TEST RESULTS?

The most agonizing hours of a medical journey are those spent waiting to hear test results. It may take hours, days, or even weeks.

Always ask how soon to expect results. The doctor or technician will give you their best estimate. That means that after the specified time has passed, you are free to call and ask for the results. Please don't call before that time, as some tests cannot be hurried, and it will only aggravate the medical personnel to keep hounding them when there's nothing they can do.

Choose how to wait.

While you and your loved one are waiting for results, you have two choices:

- Worry and get upset about the possible outcome.
- Take this time to focus on other things.

If you choose to worry about the test results, you'll only jeopardize your health, whether you're the patient, the caregiver, or a loved one. As Anglican priest William R. Inge once said, "Worry is interest paid on trouble before it comes due."[7] And according to Leo Buscaglia, PhD, "Worry never robs tomorrow of its sorrow; it only saps today of its joy."[8] Test results may affect the next step of this journey, but worrying about them will only rob you of any joy you may have today.

Taking this wait time to focus on other things will help both of you physically as well as emotionally. You both will feel calmer and side effects may diminish. And you can make positive plans for the future.

---

[7] http://thinkexist.com/quotation/worry_is_interest_paid_on_trouble_before_it_comes/227423.html

[8] http://brainyquotes.com/quotes/authors/l/leo_buscaglia_2.html

Celebrate with friends and family.

You may want to spend some time with friends and family, celebrating life and special moments with them. Take pictures. Watch fun movies. Reminisce. Laugh. We tend to be too busy with our everyday lives to take the time to find or create joy. Now would be a good time to do that.

If you're not good at coming up with ideas, find someone who is. You probably know someone who wakes up happy, laughs a lot, and always has a smile on his or her face. Chances are they know how to create joy in any circumstance. I'm one of those people, and I wouldn't mind at all if a friend asked me how to create joy while waiting for test results. It's not that hard and can be very rewarding for all involved.

At Bryan's first hospitalization, the word *cancer* came up in the doctors' conversations. So while we were waiting for Bryan's first diagnosis, we decided to create a Bucket List of things that we both wanted to do before each of us "kicked the bucket." We had already created a lot of memories, traveling and living Bryan's dream of selling his car paintings at car shows. But there were a few more things we wanted to do. Just thinking about them gave us joy for that moment and something to look forward to besides cancer and the ensuing fight.

WAITING STEP 2—SHOULD WE ASK HOW MUCH TIME WE HAVE LEFT?

Whether or not to ask about your prognosis is a personal decision, one that you may want to discuss with family and friends. It's up to each patient, along with loved ones, to decide how much information you want and what you want to do with it.

Knowing gives you control.

Many people with cancer want to know their prognosis, want to know what they're facing, and how much time they have left. Knowing will help them to complete some things that they have planned and allow them to accomplish much more than a "someday we will" approach would.

Cancer has so many unknowns. Patients and caregivers need whatever is available to help them plan treatment, make decisions, and think about lifestyle changes. Knowing what to expect, including the amount of time left, is a gift, not something to be rejected. And it's not set in stone. Bryan outlived the doctor's original expectation, but it gave us a practical way of living the time he had left. With treatment, your loved one's prognosis may change. Your oncologist can keep you posted, but you'll need to ask.

Not knowing is also a choice.

Some people choose not to know the prognosis. They'd rather not know the statistics about their cancer and or how long they have left. It's a personal choice, but one that shouldn't interfere with any preparations that must be made.

As soon as we found that Bryan's cancer was incurable, we contacted an attorney and had our wills updated. As morbid as that sounds, it saved me a lot of hassle and money, since I didn't need to go to probate court about most of our possessions. I forgot about my car and didn't have it in both of our names as Joint Tenants With Right of Survivorship (JTWROS), which meant that I needed to pay an attorney to get that car in my name alone.

Plan ahead financially.

We also discussed what Bryan wanted at his memorial service, what pictures he approved for his memorial video, and what he wanted done with his body. That made the entire process easier on me. We had the memorial service all planned before his death, so I didn't have to try to throw something together when my brain wasn't working.

Planning ahead was a blessing for both of us. I appreciated not having to start from scratch and plan a memorial service in one day. Bryan appreciated having a say in what was said and done at his service. He chose the hymns to be sung, approved pictures for the video of his life, and set the mood of the service, so he was really a part of it.

EMOTIONAL STEPS

EMOTIONAL STEP 1—
DEALING WITH ANGER

Of course you're angry. You're angry at the cancer, angry at your loved one for having cancer, angry at whatever caused this cancer, angry that your life has been interrupted, angry that your relationships have changed, angry at the caretaking you need to do, angry, angry, angry. That's to be expected. It's a normal feeling in this process.

Anger is the child of fear.

Anger is an emotion that erupts from fear. If someone is afraid of the outcome, he or she may not know how to react. Nerves are frayed and short, which can lead to angry outbursts.

If you *are* the angry one, only you can control it. No one else can. You can figure out what you're afraid of and then learn all you can about it. If you're afraid of treatment or its side effects, research to find out what you can do to make it easier and more comfortable for your loved one. If you're afraid of dying, you can get in touch with your spiritual side and learn all you can about afterlife or how to live if your loved one is gone.

If you have to live *with* an angry person, it's a little trickier. You can't stop his or her outbursts, yet you have to listen to what he or she says and live with or clean up the mess when he or she throws things. Maybe getting the person to talk will help them to see what he or she is afraid of and how to take control.

Your loved one may not know what he or she fears or even realize that he or she is afraid, so it may take some tact to get him or her to talk. You could also have a trusted friend or counselor come to visit, then leave to let them chat.

One side effect of anger is regret. You may do or say something that you'll be sorry for the rest of your life. If you stop and do the old "count to ten" when you feel the anger bubbling up, you can control your outburst.

Maybe you need some time away. Get someone to come to the house to let you leave and let the patient get away from you at the same time. Even an hour apart can rejuvenate the relationship.

Most anger grows slowly inside and then erupts when provoked. If you feel the least bit angry, take care of it right away instead of letting it fester and grow. Talk with a trusted friend, someone not directly involved in your cancer journey. Don't let it out where it can do permanent damage, but don't keep it inside, either.

Suppressed anger can show itself in physical problems. You may end up with ulcers, a digestive disorder, headaches, depression, or any number of other side effects.

Express your anger in a healthy way.

Express your anger in noncombative and nonconfrontational ways:

- Write in a journal that no one will read and then shred it.
- Paint a picture of what angers you and destroy it so no one will see it.
- Write a poem about your feelings and then tear it up.
- Get a badminton racquet and hit a mattress (while no one is on it).
- Or try any way that you know to let it out without hurting anyone.

Anger is a feeling. It's neither good nor bad. It's only bad when you express it in inappropriate ways. Do all you can to avoid letting your anger out improperly. You're worth it and so are your loved ones.

EMOTIONAL STEP 2—DOES A POSITIVE ATTITUDE REALLY HELP?

Are you one of those people who jumps out of bed in a good mood every morning and cheerfully goes about your day, no matter how boring or hard or busy it is? Most of the population doesn't wake up naturally cheerful. It's a decision that must be made every morning and many times during each day.

A positive attitude helps your body.

What difference does an attitude make? Well, your brain controls your body, keeping your heart beating, your lungs breathing, your blood pumping, and your muscles working. It's only natural that if your brain is negative, it's not running efficiently, and your machine—your body—won't run as smoothly. So elevating your brain's mood and being positive can help your body to perform at its maximum level.

According to the American Cancer Society's website, "Many people with cancer say that being told they had cancer gave them a chance to re-think their lives and find strengths and abilities that they did not know they had. Some even say that the experience has improved the quality of their lives."[9] This can be true for both patients and caregivers. Fortunately (or unfortunately), the way you cope with the rest of your life is usually the way you'll cope with your loved one's cancer. You can learn to manage differently and carry those lessons into other areas of your life.

The only true disability is a bad attitude.

---

[9] http://www.cancer.org/docroot/HOME/pff/PFF_5_1_How_Do_I_Cope.asp?sitearea=PFF

Skater and Olympic gold medal winner Scott Hamilton once said, "The only true disability in life is a bad attitude."[10] A disability is something that you must learn to work around, and a bad attitude is no different. Having to change your life for cancer is hard enough. Having others steer clear of your rotten attitude makes life that much harder. Your loved one needs a positive outlook, and you can share that.

Developing a positive attitude is not hard. Once you've chosen to be positive, it becomes easier each time until it seems natural to you. This doesn't mean that you plaster on a fake smile or put on a "plastic face." This is a change from the inside out that will revolutionize all aspects of your life.

Create a positive attitude.

Here are some basics to creating your own positive attitude:

- Take care of yourself. Give yourself permission to do something you enjoy like watching a movie, reading a book, or preparing and eating a favorite meal.
- Learn all you can about your loved one's cancer.
- Read the step in this book that explains what you're dealing with now. If you can start the day knowing what you'll face today, you can prepare for it and not be surprised.
- Express your feelings. Don't keep your emotions bottled up. Write a journal, talk with a friend, or use music, painting, or art—anything that will let you get your emotions out.
- Exercise as much as you can, even if it's just walking, yoga, or stretching, for at least 20 minutes a day.
- Reach out to others when you need help. Don't expect to travel this road alone, and don't deprive others of the opportunity to help. Your friends and loved ones want to know what they can do for you, so call and tell them.

A positive attitude can also improve the quality of your loved one's treatment and your relationships. We all know someone whose bad attitude or cynicism made him or her difficult to be around for any length of time. Health care professionals and friends are no different in that respect than we are.

---

[10] *http://brainyquotes.com/quotes/authors/s/scott_hamilton_2.html*

A positive attitude can result in better care.

Bryan and I discovered that having a pleasant outlook made his nurses and doctors enjoy the time they spent with us, so they took their time and stayed with us as long as we wanted them there. Our hospice chaplain said he looked forward to visiting us, as our home had such a pleasant air about it. And many friends came to visit for a "joy fix" from us. Had we been angry or bitter, we may have spent more time alone, time when we needed people around.

Staying hopeful can improve the quality of your life, whether or not you have cancer. You can't cure cancer with a positive attitude, but you can make every day more bearable and improve your life. Don't expect to always be upbeat. You will feel sad, stressed, anxious, a variety of emotions along this journey. This is normal, but staying mentally positive can help keep those emotions under control.

EMOTIONAL STEP 3—BEING THANKFUL

I'm caring for a loved one with cancer! What do I have to be thankful for? That's asking a lot, wanting me to be thankful for something as horrible as cancer when life was hard enough already.

Here's where a positive attitude can make a big difference. And thankfulness will help develop that attitude. If you can look at the plus side of things, you'll see that there are some advantages:

- Your priorities have finally come into focus. You realize what's really important and what's fluff.
- Your family and friends want to help you and won't mind if you ask. In fact, they may drop everything to help you.

Point out the positive!

You can point out some positive things to your loved one:

- Your health care team is focused on his or her healing and comfort.
- Medical science has made dramatic advances recently, and this cancer is likely to respond to treatment.
- He or she doesn't have the urge to overeat.
- Neither one of you has the time or energy to run up credit card bills.
- Others will forgive both of you for a snit of anger.
- Your loved one can eat all he or she wants.
- Your loved one can sleep all he or she wants.
- His or her drugs are legal.

OK, a few of those are a little flippant, but if you try hard enough, you can find many things to be thankful for just like I did. Write them down, even if they make you smile—especially if they make you smile. Add to your list whenever you think of something else. Read your list often to remind yourself of all that you're thankful for. Then, give yourself permission to be appreciative.

Your attitude is totally up to you, so you can decide to be grateful for what you have (love, family, and friends) and what you don't have (worse problems). It helps to take your mind off what you're facing and give it a positive spin.

EMOTIONAL STEP 4—WE'RE AFRAID

Fear is normal. It's what keeps us from things that might hurt us. It keeps us from running onto a busy highway, touching a live electric wire, or jumping into the lion's cage at the zoo. We know the likely consequences, so we avoid them.

Fear is normal.

Fear in the cancer journey, however, is usually fear of the unknown. You don't know how treatment will work, how long it will take, what side effects your loved one will have, how people will change toward you, whether your loved one will die, what death is, and any number of other things.

Another word for fear is *anxiety*. You're anxious or uneasy. That's normal, considering the circumstances. No one would expect or think any less of you, and they'd be surprised if you weren't anxious or afraid.

Fear can show itself in angry outbursts. In the episode titled "Moon" of the long-running television series *Touched by an Angel*, Monica the angel, in talking to someone who was always angry, stated, "Anger is the child of fear."[11] That means that angry people are afraid of something but don't know how to face their fear. They react in anger, which can appear as yelling, snippy comebacks, "the silent treatment," a short temper over little things, and many other unpleasant interactions. The age-old "Well, *excu-u-u-use* me!" was on the tip of my tongue many times during Bryan's illness, but I knew it would hurt, so I never said it. It wasn't easy, but I didn't want to live with that regret.

Find someone to talk with.

The hardest part in dealing with fear is figuring out what you're afraid of or anxious about. It helps if you have someone with whom you can talk openly. This may be difficult for a patient and caregiver to discuss with each

---

[11] http://www.jenniofshalott.net/tbaa/allquotes.html

other. Usually, the caregiver is a spouse or close family member who may be hurt if the patient bares his or her soul. The caregiver may feel that the sacrifice and work aren't appreciated, or the caregiver may be afraid as well and not want to be open with the patient, adding to the pain.

Find a third party, maybe a close friend or counselor, someone you can trust not to reveal your deepest, darkest secrets. That may be difficult, especially for a man, but it's not impossible. A nurse or hospice employee may be able to help and listen.

Bryan and I talked regularly about our emotions, but he was afraid of hurting me by telling me his true gut feelings. I received a phone call one day when our visiting nurse was here, so I was distracted and in another room for a while. Bryan opened up to Keitha, whom he trusted, and thanked her profusely for listening and just letting him talk.

Learn all you can.

Another way of handling fear is to learn all you can. As the saying goes, "Knowledge is power," so educate yourself. Just using this book can give you some power and control over what's happening.

The first thing you need to learn is what type of cancer you and your loved one are fighting, what ammunition you have, and how to fight. You can do like I did and search the web. The chapter in this book titled, "Information Step 2—Where can I find more information?" will give some details, but be sure you're on a reputable site. Anyone can create a website and post whatever they want, so you can't always trust everything you read.

You can also visit a library or a bookstore for information. Be warned: Most cancer books either cover only the most common cancers or try to include every possible cancer topic. You may get too much book to digest, so try to find precise, useful information.

You may discover that your brain isn't as sharp as usual, and you can't grasp what you're reading. That's normal. Don't beat yourself up. You already have so many things going through your head that you may be on information overload. Read what you can, when you can, and take notes so you can read those later. You won't remember everything, but you can remember enough to give you the confidence you need.

Explore your spirituality.

Another thing that creates fear is the possibility of death. Even though it's a normal, natural stage of life, death can seem ominous because of its finality. Everyone has a spiritual side, and you need to explore yours if you haven't already.

Find answers to questions such as:

- What do you believe about life and death?
- Is there life after death?
- What happens when you stop breathing?

Bryan and I were blessed to be in families that believed in God and everlasting life, offered by the death and resurrection of Jesus Christ. So when Bryan found himself at death's door, he was ready to take that last step. In fact, at the end he became upset when people prayed for his healing. He said, "Once we accept Christ into our lives, we are always looking forward to being with him in heaven. Now that I'm on the doorstep, some people won't let me go!"

Believing in God is easy. He exists whether we believe or not, so the choice to believe is up to me. I just need to admit the world doesn't revolve around me and that there is a greater power, an intelligent being in charge. It gave Bryan and me such peace, knowing that God is in charge and knew what we were facing. He welcomed Bryan home when his journey here was done.

If you want that kind of assurance, call or visit a church near you and ask them to explain God's plan of salvation to you. If they can't, try another church. You've made an informed decision about your treatment, so why not make an informed decision about your life?

Find heaven experiences at *www.SeeHope.com*.

For more specific information, you can check out the website of my editor and friend, Hope Flinchbaugh, at *www.SeeHope.com*. She has interviewed people who have "died" and gone to heaven, however briefly, and lived to tell about it. She also has a link to explain how to get to heaven.

Another way to find out is to get a New Testament and start reading. You can skip to the Book of John, if you want to avoid all the "begats" in Matthew. Either one will explain the life of Jesus and how it can impact you.

Latch on to peace.

It's up to you to decide what you believe, what gives you peace, and the assurance that death isn't the end. The French philosopher and Nobel Prize winner Albert Camus said, "I would rather live my life as if there is a God and die to find out there isn't, than live my life as if there isn't and die to find out there is."[12] Rest assured that there is a God, and he loves you, no matter what you believe about him.

Knowing there is a God and life after death can give you peace that others don't understand. It's important at this stage. Not believing or accepting him is totally up to you.

---

[12] http://brainyquotes.com/quotes/authors/a/albert_camus_2.html

EMOTIONAL STEP 5—NO REGRETS

Start doing today what you've meant to do for so long. Start today. It's that simple. Start now. Don't delay any longer. Bryan and I had created many memories before he was diagnosed. We traveled, visited with family, lived Bryan's dream of selling his car paintings at car shows, and did so many things that people tend to put off until "later" or "someday." Do what you can today to create good memories for tomorrow.

List things you want to do.

Make a list of things that you have wanted to do, a sort of "bucket list," then do them if and when you can. When our boys were little, we would sit down as a family and each of us in turn would say one thing they'd like to do or a place they'd like to go. This might include McDonald's, Disney World, ice skating, Dairy Queen, or whatever we could think up. This was brainstorming, so nothing was off limits, and all suggestions were written down. We'd go around the circle until we were out of ideas. Then we would hang the list on the refrigerator. When we had an hour to do an activity, time to go out to dinner, or a vacation to plan, we'd look at the list to see what we could accomplish, then cross it off the list.

Start your list today. Write down anything you'd like to do, no matter how crazy it may seem. You'll be surprised how it can lift your spirits, just thinking of hopes and dreams. Then add to your list whenever you think of something else. If and when you can, do something on the list and check it off. This will give you something to anticipate and moments to remember.

What you can do today.

Here are some things you can do now to avoid regrets later:

- Be more patient than usual. It isn't easy, but it's worth it.
- Reminisce on good times.

- Spend as much time together as possible. No one ever wished they had spent more time working than with family and loved ones.
- Go through old photographs together and share memories.
- Laugh together. Watch funny movies or situation comedies on television.
- Read to each other. Let children read to you.
- Follow the great commandment, "Do unto others as you would have them do unto you." Imagine what it would be like to be your loved one, and try to sense what he or she feels.
- Be conscious of how you treat each other.
- Stop and think before you react in anger. Count to ten.
- Enjoy your time together as much as possible.
- Ask what your loved one needs, then get it for him or her, the best you can.

Life is hard enough without having to regret choices we made in the past, especially at this important stage in your life. It's time now to do something different, and it's up to you. Just do it.

EMOTIONAL STEP 6—WHAT IS GRIEF?

Even if you've just gotten the diagnosis, you're grieving. No one has died, but you're grieving what you've lost forever: good health, the bliss of ignorance, your "normal" life, and the way things used to be.

Elisabeth Kübler-Ross introduced the five stages of grief in 1969 in her book *On Death and Dying*:[13]

Denial

This is when you can't believe what is happening. You may temporarily pretend that nothing has changed and that life will go on unaffected, one day at a time. You have probably gone past this stage since you're reading this book and are dealing with reality.

Anger

This is where you scream and yell, "It's not fair!" "Why us?" "Who or what is to blame for this?" It's OK to feel the anger, but be careful that you don't inflict permanent damage to yourself or your relationships. See "Emotional Step 1—Dealing with anger" for tips on how to control this feeling.

Denial-Anger-Bargaining-Depression-Acceptance

Bargaining

This stage can come at any time in the journey. You start wondering if you or your loved one could have or should have done something different or if you can do something differently now. Maybe you could have altered the outcome or stopped the cancer from ever coming. Maybe if you change

---

[13] http://grief.com/the-five-stages-of-grief/

something now, it will go away. This is the "What if..." game. It doesn't hurt to think of all the possibilities, but don't let them ruin your life.

Depression

Depression

This is the low point. Many of us have been there before, and it's not where we want to spend our lives. Talking with a loved one or a counselor or getting help from your doctor can reduce the extent of this stage.

Acceptance

You realize what's happening and prepare to fight and do whatever is necessary. You tell yourself that everything will be OK and you can handle the outcome.

These steps don't always come in the same order. You may need to repeat one or more, and you may experience two at the same time, but they will all make an appearance. If you know they're coming, you can prepare for them and handle them better than if you're blindsided.

RELATIONSHIP STEPS

RELATIONSHIP STEP 1—
WHO DO WE TELL? AND HOW?

Tell anyone who cares. People care—probably more people than you realize, and not just family. They want you both to do well and to be well, and they're concerned when you're not. Let them share in your journey.

When Bryan first became ill, I called or e-mailed only those who needed notification that we wouldn't be at a meeting, a rehearsal, a party, or work. Eventually, the e-mails were more about Bryan's condition than the fact that we would miss a previously planned get-together. That's when the number of recipients grew.

Friends and family members forwarded my e-mails to others they knew who were going through similar experiences. They wanted my words to help their loved ones on their cancer journeys. Many of these "friends of friends" became my friends, and contacted me personally to ask questions, request parts of my book, or ask to be added to my distribution list.

This is a road best traveled with friends.

I was thrilled— and I'm still thrilled— to help anyone who finds himself or herself in the role of cancer caregiver or patient. This is a road best traveled with friends. That's why I have a blog where you can contact me directly with your questions, hopes, fears, dreams, or whatever is on your mind. Look for me at *SteppingThroughCancer.com*. I included the first chapter of this book downloadable from this site, too, for anyone who just received a cancer diagnosis and is not sure where to turn. Send them here!

You don't need to call each person in your address book and spend hours on the phone repeating the same things over and over. I made that mistake when my husband had a serious car accident. I practically lived at the hospital for the eight days he was there and ran up our cell phone bill in the process.

You also don't need to e-mail each person or reply to each message individually. That's another mistake I made. On the days I went home to sleep instead of dozing in the chair by his hospital bed, I spent hours on the computer, keeping me from his side that much longer. I would e-mail one person, copy and paste it into a new message, modify the message to personalize it for the new recipient, and then resend it. Talk about time-consuming!

Spreading the News By E-Mail

I finally came up with the best way to spread the news: mass e-mail. I wrote one e-mail and sent it to friends and family near and far, asking them to forward it to anyone I may have missed. Using the same method when Bryan had cancer, the one hundred people I e-mailed were forwarding to several hundred more, so that we eventually had a thousand readers and prayer warriors.

One drawback to e-mail is that you may have a limited number of addressees allowed for each message. I can only send to one hundred recipients at a time; any more, and the e-mail won't go anywhere.

Here is the best way to keep track of your recipients, especially when you have over a hundred people who want to receive your e-mails directly:

Open a new spreadsheet file on your computer. Be sure to save it in a folder you can locate later for revisions. In Column A, list all the people you want to contact. Copy and paste each e-mail address from your e-mail address book into Column B.

In Column C, add a word or two indicating how you know the person: church, work, family, car club, or whatever. Then sort the list by Column C, and you'll have different groups to e-mail.

Go back to the contact list in your e-mail and create an e-mail group for each group you had sorted. Give each group a name, such as "Update Church" or "Update Family."

When you send one e-mail to everyone you want to contact at work or at church, the recipients can see who already got the message. They can then forward it on to others not in the group who might be interested as well. That way, you'll reach more than the hundred that you might contact personally.

There are multiple web-based services that will work as well. If you're already active in a method of contacting friends, use that one since you already have readers. But don't forget non-techie folks who have no e-mail or computer. You can have someone send them a paper copy or have someone set up a phone tree to call each one individually. That way, you don't have to make all those calls.

To be sure your message will be read and forwarded, be sure to make it:

- Informative.
- Precise (not too wordy).
- Upbeat.

Keep your general reports and messages upbeat.

People are much more likely to read and forward a message that gives hope or encouragement, especially if the message is from someone facing a seemingly hopeless situation. They're also more likely to reach out and help you if you're not all down in the dumps. Encouragement is contagious, so learn it and pass it along.

You may not feel hopeful or encouraged as you write. In fact, you may feel the exact opposite: despondent, depressed, and hopeless. Everyone would understand if you felt that way, but they would come to dread your e-mails if the messages contained only doom and gloom, no matter how much they loved you.

Writing about hope and joy will help you as well as your readers.

If you write about hope and joy instead, you'll be surprised how remarkable your messages will be, for you as well as for your readers. As you look for something positive to add to each e-mail, you will discover a positive attitude within you, making your journey more bearable.

Bryan and I had learned to look for what we called "the point of the story" in movies and TV shows. Someone will usually say something poignant at a critical moment that puts the entire story in a nutshell. When we'd hear a line like that, we'd point at the screen, meaning that was the point of the story. Those points usually put a positive spin on the situation in the story. Those points ended up being my words of hope or encouragement.

E-Mail Examples

Here are some examples from the e-mails I sent:

- July 29, after Bryan's PET scan, where we saw multiple tumors: *While in the many waiting rooms and hospital rooms, I've been reading* The Lord of the Rings *trilogy. One thing I read today jumped off the page. For those who don't know, Frodo has been charged with a difficult task of returning the Ring, and going through some really tough situations to complete his mission: "'I am commanded to go to the land of Mordor, and therefore I shall go,' said Frodo. 'If there is only one way, then I must take it. What comes after must come.'"[14] I guess that's the way it is for all of us. If this is what we must do, then we just do it, whatever comes. I guess this is what Bryan and I do for now.*

- August 1, after we received the final diagnosis that Bryan's cancer was not treatable: *I was listening to AM 910 this morning, and they played a song by Steven Curtis Chapman called "The Miracle of the Moment." The chorus goes something like this:*

  > *There's a wonder in the here and now*
  > *It's right there in front of you*
  > *And I don't want you to miss*
  > *The miracle of the moment* [15]

  We decided that will be our goal now, to look for the miracle in each moment we have, since we don't know how many moments are left. We hope you do the same. We all spend so much time looking forward to "special" moments that we miss how special this moment is. Enjoy today's moments!

This is a tough journey, and others will want to help.

---

[14] Tolkien, John Ronald Reuel, *THE TWO TOWERS: Being the Second Part of The Lord of the Rings Trilogy*. Random House, Inc., 2001, p. 273.

[15] "The Miracle Of The Moment," words and music by Steven Curtis Chapman and Matt Bronleewe. Used by permission.

Even in life's darkest times, you can still find hope and encouragement; you just have to look a little harder than usual. Keep reading mail, newspapers, books, magazines, or whatever interests you. Something will jump out at you, begging to be shared. It may make a difference in you as well.

When you watch television or a movie, keep paper and pen handy, so you can jot down those "Aha!" moments, the comments or statements that make your mind click. You think you'll remember them, but that's asking a lot of your brain, especially now. Write them down so you can read them later. They'll stay with you longer and have a stronger impact on you and your readers.

I heard of one family who did something as simple as recording a daily incoming message on their answering machine and having everyone call their home to listen to the latest update. That way, they could ignore the phone and not have to repeat the information over and over.

Find what works for you and do it. This is a tough journey, and others will want to help. Keep them informed and involved.

RELATIONSHIP STEP 2— WILL PRAYER HELP?

Will prayer help? Absolutely!

The more people you can enlist as your prayer warriors, the better. When Bryan was ill, we had not only the members of our own church praying, but also family and friends across the country. I was e-mailing regular updates, reaching about a thousand people. Many told us that they put Bryan on their church's prayer lists, so there were even more prayers.

Knowing that others care, are thinking of me, and are sharing my requests with the God of the universe assures me that I am not alone. My relationship with Christ permeates my entire life, so having another connection and an intercessor in times of trouble always helps me. It can help you as well.

Prayer is proven effective in scientific studies.

Although many consider prayer a religious thing, many studies have been done to determine if it makes a difference in one's health or healing. Prayer can make a difference even if the patient doesn't know that he or she has been prayed for.

The National Center for Complementary and Alternative Medicine (NCCAM), a part of the U.S. government's National Institutes of Health, reported in their Winter 2005 newsletter that prayer was the most common therapy used by patients.

Catherine Stoney, Ph.D., a program officer in NCCAM's Division of Extramural Research and Training, pointed to evidence of a connection between prayer and health outcomes. She stated there was "evidence that religious affiliation and religious practices are associated with health and mortality—in other words, with better health and longer life. Such connections may involve immune function, cardiovascular function, and/or other physiological changes."[16]

---

[16] CAM at the NIH, National Center for Complementary and Alternative Medicine, found at *http://nccam.nih.gov/news/newsletter/CAMatNIH.htm*

Dr. Stoney noted that religious practice may be an effective way of coping with stress, which in itself can have beneficial health effects. It's no secret that those with a religious outlook on life tend to live longer, more satisfying lives. Knowing that there is an all-knowing Creator in charge and things aren't just left to chance can eliminate a lot of anxiety, which in turn may result in better health.

Prayer affects patients positively.

Dr. Mitch Krucoff, professor of medicine and cardiology at Duke University Medical Center, directs the cardiovascular devices unit at Duke Clinical Research Institute. He has performed several studies to determine the effect prayer has on patients. While results of prayed-for and non-prayed-for groups were similar, a survey after one study indicated that most of the patients believed they were in the prayed-for group. That alone may indicate the power of prayer: a patient had only to *think* someone was praying for him or her to get positive health benefits!

Some people feel that praying is just "mumbo-jumbo." In fact, a professional psychologist told my teenage son those words during a counseling session, which upset my son and us very much. Just because you disagree with someone's religious belief doesn't mean you can shoot them down or belittle their belief system. Be respectful of the patient's and the family's religious beliefs.

When friends wanted to come and pray for Bryan's healing, they asked first for our permission. We allowed them and were thankful that they had given us the option, not forcing their belief system on us.

Although Bryan's cancer was untreatable, many prayers helped both of us in our attitudes, giving us much-needed peace and comfort. Those prayers supported me and made it possible for me to survive and grow from the experience. For me, prayer always helps.

RELATIONSHIP STEP 3—SHOULD WE ACCEPT VISITORS?

Visitors can either brighten your day or make it unbearable. You can usually tell before they come which effect they'll have and choose accordingly. The decision of which visitors to admit is mainly up to the patient, but the caregiver is normally the one on the phone making arrangements.

Some visitors must be allowed in. These may be family members or health care professionals, including hospice volunteers, counselors, chaplains or religious leaders, or others helping in the journey. To deny them access to the patient may be detrimental to the patient's health and relationships.

Positive Visits

Having cancer may give you time to visit with those important to you, mend or build relationships, and finally say what needs to be said. Take advantage of this opportunity. Bryan's son Gene visited several times from out of state, giving them time to cement their father-son bond and work through some things that had been clouding their relationship for years. Bryan was pleased each time Gene came to visit, and slept well after each conversation.

Turning Away Visitors

Other visitors can be tactfully turned away, especially if the patient would be upset by their visit. Even a family member can be difficult to handle, particularly one who doesn't live in the area or has not visited a lot. Having him or her appear on the doorstep when you're having trouble dealing with day-to-day life may be more than both of you can handle.

Small children could disrupt the household, mainly because they can make a lot of noise and expend a lot of energy when the patient needs peace and quiet. As hard as it may be, you may need to tell some friends or family members not to visit or that they can come only if their children do not.

Feeling ill is a valid reason to deny a request to visit. It's also a perfect excuse if someone calls to schedule a visit and you would rather not see them. They'll understand.

When the patient isn't feeling well, disruptions can be very upsetting. Bryan preferred listening to quiet "elevator music" and dozing whenever possible rather than having to sit up and be sociable. When he would lie down during a visit, I knew the conversation was over and asked our visitor to leave. Some days, Bryan would ask me to cancel a visit because he wanted to sleep.

Who May Visit

When friends or family would call to see if they could visit, Bryan's litmus test was whether they had visited our home within the past three years. As he lost weight, he was uncomfortable having people stare at him. He stated on many occasions, "If they didn't care enough to visit before, now that I'm a cancer 'freak' I don't want them coming to see the 'freak show.'" I had to respect that decision and turn away some visitors that I would have liked to see, just because it would have been uncomfortable for Bryan.

If out-of-town visitors are coming, decide whether you want them to stay at your house or at a nearby hotel. If they stay with you, limit their visit to just a few days. The patient will try to be "up" and sociable during the visit, which can be very strenuous. Having Bryan's best friend, Ken, in the house was great for me, since Bryan trusted him and I could leave them alone in the house for a few hours to go shopping. However, I didn't keep his visit short, and Bryan was ready for him to leave after a few days.

Not everyone who calls needs to be coming to spend time with the patient. The caregiver needs support as well, and can take a visitor to a different room while the patient sleeps. My good friend Allison visited every Friday afternoon, bringing a Village Inn pie with her, sharing experiences of her and her husband's cancer journeys with me, and informing me what to anticipate. This was invaluable in helping me cope and letting me know I could get through this.

How To Handle Drop-Ins

Most people will be courteous and call first. But some folks will just drop by without warning. That doesn't obligate you to let them in if it's not a good time. Some friends arrived once while our hospice doctor was here. There was no way we could have them in the room while we were carrying on a private conversation. They understood once it was explained, thanked us, and left. Our relationship was unharmed.

There are a lot of variables that need to be considered about visitors, the most important of which is, *Is this good for the patient?* Ask yourself this question every time someone calls or comes to visit.

You don't need to give in to everyone else's requests. Just decide if it's right or not. It's up to you.

RELATIONSHIP STEP 4—HOW DO
WE RECORD MEMORIES?

Start with a camera. Take pictures, lots of pictures. If you have a video camera, use it, and don't forget to record voices, favorite songs, or any sounds you hear, even if only on a tape recorder or on your phone.

Take pictures.

A picture is truly worth a thousand words, so take pictures of your guests, alone and with the patient. It will then be easier for you to remember your visitors and the good times you had. If possible, audibly record their visits (especially if it's your pastor or a chaplain) with their permission, of course. Their encouraging words can bear repeating.

As you get your prints, assemble them in a box or a notebook so you can flip through them whenever you want to reminisce. You don't need to spend a lot of time or money making creative photo albums. Just put the pictures in a box or a book so you can look at them and remember.

After my sister Barb passed away, her daughter Patti and I were remembering her and the fun times we had. Patti had taken a picture of her mom just a short while before, when Barb had insisted on eating the flower on her birthday cake made of dark blue icing. Then, when Patti took her smiling picture and posted it on Facebook, her blue lips and teeth were immortalized and brought laughter to an otherwise sad time.

Talk and record memories.

Take time talking with your loved one and anyone else and then recording those memories, no matter how trivial. If you don't put them on paper or another medium, you'll forget them.

Before Gramma Mac passed away at the age of 99, we gave her a small book with questions to record her memories on paper. There were questions about her schooling, when cars first arrived in her town, her first telephone, where she had her first date, and other memories that only she would have.

It would have been a wonderful resource, but she never wrote in it. Instead of just giving her the book, we should have taken time with her, asking the questions and writing the answers as she gave them.

One of the best gifts I ever gave was the photo album for my son Brian's twenty-fifth birthday, covering his first quarter-century. He spent the next half-hour sharing the pictures and his memories with his girlfriend and his grandmother, accompanied by lots of smiles and laughter. Your memories can do the same.

RELATIONSHIP STEP 5—ASKING FOR AND RECEIVING HELP

Some people believe that asking for help is a sign of weakness. But when you and your loved one are battling cancer, asking for help is a way to let your friends and family become allies in your fight. You don't have to fight alone.

Why Ask for Help?

If you ask for help:

- You can save your energy for more important things.
- The patient will feel less guilty about being a burden to you, the caregiver.
- Others may be able to do things better or more easily.

Many friends and family members will offer help with the usual, "Let me know if you need anything." They have no idea what you want or need, so have in mind a few things you can ask them for.

Ways Family and Friends Can Help

Here are some specific ways friends and family can help you:

- **Providing meals.** We received many frozen meals that we could heat and eat at our convenience. Let them know what you and your loved one enjoy eating and especially if there's a food item your loved one really can't have.
- **Cleaning house.** Attacking a dirty bathroom was the last thing I wanted to do. Some friends spent one afternoon cleaning house for us; my son Brian and his wife, Sarah, cleaned for us another time.
- **Children.** Let someone take care of them to give you some rest.

- **Shopping.** A friend who lived nearby would call when she was heading to the grocery store to see if we needed anything. Keep a shopping list handy so you can be specific.
- **Yard work.** If you don't want to get dirty, let someone else do it. If you really love it, ask someone to stay in the house with your loved one for an hour or two, since you may not hear the patient call if you're outside.
- **Letting you talk.** Both patient and caregiver need some time away from each other and the opportunity to talk openly.
- **Gathering information.** You don't need to do all the research yourself. Others are computer-literate and want to help.
- **Driving.** When I was working at the office, Bryan's daughter would take him to doctors' appointments.

When someone offers help, don't be shy. They want to help, so give them the opportunity.

Some May Refuse

Be aware that some people may refuse for various reasons:

- This may be a bad time for them. It doesn't mean that they won't ever help, just not now. They may be dealing with their own problems.
- They may not know how to help. You can be specific, for example, "I just can't face cleaning the toilet. Can you please do that for me?" This worked for me.
- They may be uncomfortable around someone who is sick. One dear friend apologized for not coming, but she insisted that she was weak and couldn't visit. Instead, she sent encouraging e-mails that helped me to cope.

Don't judge anyone who can't help right now. They mean well, but may not be able to handle it right now. Let it go.

Most people want to help. Don't deny them the privilege. They want to know that you and they did everything possible, so let them. It's a gift you can give that costs you nothing and repays immensely.

And it's something they want to offer.

RELATIONSHIP STEP 6—FAMILY CAN BE UGLY, ESPECIALLY WHEN YOU LEAST EXPECT IT

Some people have trouble dealing with difficulty, and they may create more problems than you are prepared to deal with. Unfortunately, this may come from a family member who should be offering support instead of trouble.

Some individuals don't know what to say and end up saying the wrong thing. A friend told me about a lady whose sister was fighting cancer. Instead of expressing sympathy, she told her sister, "I'm glad you have cancer and not me." This may have seemed harmless to the speaker, but it was devastating to the patient. The wrong words can ruin a relationship if we let them.

When Someone Says the Wrong Thing

If possible, tactfully let him or her know that what was said hurt, and maybe he or she will apologize. If he or she is unable to apologize, let it go. Life is too precious to waste time feeling wounded by insensitive fools. You may need to refuse to let the person visit, for fear of more insensitivity and needless pain. If you need it, you now have permission to keep that person from visiting.

Family members not directly involved in day-to-day decisions and treatment may second-guess your actions. They may hear of a "wonder treatment" and want you to try it, no matter how strange it sounds. If you don't at least try their ideas, they may blame you for years to come. Thank them politely for their suggestions, but assure them that you, your loved one, and your oncologist have investigated all possibilities and are following the best treatment plan.

> **Loved ones are in pain, too.**

Some loved ones may feel that the caregiver doesn't do enough. They may become distant or show their anger after the patient's death. This type of action is a result of grief stuck in the bargaining stage—they can only think "what if" or "if only" instead of reality. A friend of mine has no contact with her husband's family because they repeatedly accused her of not doing enough to keep him alive. Actually, she had dedicated herself to his care for months and did all that was humanly possible.

Some may decide that this is the time to resolve old grudges. If possible, and it won't upset the patient, let them. It may be good for all concerned. But keep the patient's wishes in mind when you allow visitors. If your loved one would be uncomfortable with a certain family member, politely deny that family member's request to come.

> **You decide who to talk to and visit with.**

You have some say in who visits and who communicates by phone. If someone is hurtful, you can ask the person to leave, ask him or her not to come back, or even hang up on the person if he or she is unkind on the telephone. It's your life and your home. You decide what's good for you and your loved one. This time is too valuable for you to waste on prickly relationships.

Family can help immensely at this time. They can also inflict pain. Be wary of the latter, as you have enough pain already.

RELATIONSHIP STEP 7—DEALING WITH ISSUES LONG-DISTANCE

Some people have the misfortune of being miles away from their loved one with cancer and having to manage things from a distance. While this isn't easy, it can be done.

Most communication will be by telephone or e-mail, but it's tough to assess real needs without being there in person. The patient can give the answers he or she thinks you want to hear without telling you how he or she really feels. Try to read between the lines or hear what's not being said. The more you converse openly, the more you can recognize his or her tone and tell when something changes, like pain levels. You will need to judge if something can be dealt with from a distance or if it will require an in-person visit.

Build a local support network.

Build a local support network for your loved one, comprised of both paid and volunteer workers including friends and church members. Record all their names and numbers, noting those who will accept a call from you day or night or in a crisis. A local phone book from your loved one's area will give you access to other resources and may be easier to navigate than a web-based directory.

Contact your telephone service provider to see if they have any way of reducing your long-distance bill, such as a package plan with lower toll rates. Many cell phones have unlimited or free long-distance calling, or you may consider purchasing a prepaid phone card with a lower rate.

Share your home, work, and cell phone numbers with health care providers and others involved. They may need to contact you in an emergency.

You may want to stay in contact via computer. A local family member or friend can create a blog or website to post daily updates. Talk with a computer expert about any new ways to communicate using video and audio. Technology advances are always presenting new ways of communicating that make it easier to stay in touch. Don't be afraid to try something new.

Check for travel deals.

Contact a travel agent to see if there are any special deals for patients or family members. A social worker at the hospital or with hospice may know of other resources, such as private pilots or companies who would help. When my brother Ken needed transportation, a friend with a small airplane flew him and his wife cross-country free of charge to a university cancer center.

If you travel, be sure to schedule time to rest when you return. Your visit will be demanding, and travel is always strenuous, so give yourself time to relax before you have to get back to your daily grind.

Long-distance care is difficult, but not impossible. Create a local support system to do the things that you would do if you were there in person. And give yourself permission to travel as much as needed. You don't want to live with the regret of not doing everything possible.

STEPS YOU WANTED TO KNOW ABOUT BUT WERE AFRAID TO ASK

STEP 1—PREPARING FOR THE WORST, BELIEVING THE BEST

Death is a natural part of life, but most people are afraid of it and make the mistake of ignoring it. Preparing for it will make the transition easier for all involved, and isn't as gloomy as you may think. Knowing that the details for the surviving family members are taken care of will reassure the patient and relieve stress for all involved.

Update Your Wills

The most important step is to prepare or update your will. Both patient and caregiver should do this. When we were updating Bryan's will, the lawyer prepared my will at the same time for the same fee, saving us money.

Be specific about what you want each person to receive. Don't just leave everything for your children to divide. If you do, everything will need to be valued and divided evenly or sold. When one wants your living room television and another wants your sofa, specify both so there is no question of who gets what. Many a family has been torn apart or ended up in court over an unclear will. No one really wants to sell your antique tea set and split the proceeds, so be precise.

Meet With a Financial Adviser

Meet with a financial planner or adviser. It may be too late to get a life insurance policy for the patient, but you can be sure everything else is in order. Your financial adviser can keep track of your funds and maybe put them into protected accounts so that a poor economy won't significantly affect you.

This may be the time to think about getting life insurance for yourself. It's not as expensive as you think, and it will help your loved ones in the event of your death. Money can't buy love, happiness, or an extended life, but it can make the details of life and preparing for death much easier.

JTWROS on All Cars

If you and your spouse own cars jointly, be sure the ownership on each title is Joint Tenants with Right of Survivorship (JTWROS). That means that if one of you dies, the other automatically has sole ownership of the car. Without JTWROS, you can't get the title changed to just one name unless a probate judge orders it, which can cost you time and money. You can't sell the car until it is only in the name of the survivor.

Power of Attorney

A power of attorney allows a spouse to sign papers in the other's name, but only as long as the other is alive. Be sure your attorney has looked at all your legal papers so ownership will transfer without complications.

Sign and Date Papers

Sign any necessary papers and date them. If you need a notary, you can find one through your bank or on the internet. If you're unable to go to them, call to see if they can come to your home. They may require a nominal fee for their service, whether at their location or yours.

Know All About Bills

Make sure someone knows about all the bills including monthly utilities, rent or mortgage, Home Owners Association fees, and any other monthly, biannual, or annual bills you have. Also, gather information on checking and savings accounts. It helps if you can set up a file or drawer to keep track of what's been paid and what's still due. These will need to be paid during your cancer journey, so you may want to have someone else take over for now. This may require a power of attorney if the payer's name isn't on the checking account. Too often, spouses are in the dark when the patient was the bill-payer and didn't reveal his or her system.

Write Down Your Loved One's Wishes

Write down your loved one's desires about his or her care, and be sure you and every other caregiver know them. This will include under what conditions he or she wishes to be resuscitated, how he or she wants pain meds administered, who will make medical decisions when he or she cannot, and other situations. Aging With Dignity, a nonprofit organization, produces *Five Wishes*, a booklet that allows the patient to be specific about what they want to happen.

The Five Wishes include:

1. Who can make decisions when the patient cannot.
2. Allowed medical treatment.
3. Managing comfort.
4. How the patient wants to be treated.
5. What the patient wants loved ones to know.

This booklet is available at *www.agingwithdignity.org* or through your hospital or health care provider. I would advise you and your loved one to each prepare your wishes. If you want to write your own, be as specific as possible about the items above. Give copies to your grown children and to your health care organization, so they will have it on file. Bryan and I had prepared our Five Wishes after a serious car accident two years before his cancer diagnosis, so we were set in advance.

Write Instructions for the Family

Write a letter of instructions as a guide for yourself and the family. This isn't a legal document, but it will have a list of names and numbers of people your loved one wants contacted, locations of important papers, whom you want to take your loved one's pets, if applicable, and what kind of funeral or memorial service your loved one wants.

Give copies of this letter to the executor of your and your loved one's wills, your family, and other loved ones. They need to know what kind of service you want before they plan it, and whom to contact right away.

The thing to remember is the old Boy Scout motto, "Be prepared." It makes the journey much easier if everyone is prepared for whatever may come.

STEP 2—WHAT IS A COMA?
SHOULD WE EXPECT IT?

Coma is a form of unconsciousness where the patient appears to be sleeping. Your loved one may or may not have to deal with coma in his or her journey. Talk with your health care providers to see if this is something you'll face. Bryan's cancer was in the bile ducts that drain his liver, so he slipped into a hepatic coma, meaning liver failure, and "slept" for seven days.

Levels of Consciousness

There are differing levels of consciousness while in a coma. The patient's eyes are almost always closed, so he or she probably won't see anything. However, the patient may be able to hear what is going on around him or her.

I was told that if Bryan cried out when I tried to move him, insert pain meds, or touch him in any way, the pain would subside just as quickly. I found a better way: If I warned Bryan of what I was going to do, he would cooperate without a sound. All I had to say was, "Bryan, I'm going to lift your legs to straighten the sheets," and he would lie there quietly and let me do whatever I needed to do.

He also could hear and understand what I said to him while comatose. Bryan had always been particular about his teeth, so I continued brushing them when he couldn't do it any longer. When he was in a coma and I told him I wanted to brush his teeth, he would relax his jaw and open his mouth enough to insert a toothbrush. Then, when I told him I was done, he would close his mouth again and go back to sleep.

> **Keep trying until you figure out what they need!**

I also discovered that Bryan could feel physical discomfort and could communicate with me. On the fifth day of his coma, he appeared to be trying to talk with me and with his daughter Lisa. He scrunched up his nose and moved his lips like he was saying the letter W. We opened the drapes thinking he wanted to look out the window; we offered him water through a straw; and we tried everything we could think of that began with a W. I finally realized that his moustache hadn't been trimmed and was tickling his nose! After a trim, he settled down and went back to sleep.

If the coma is drug-induced, the patient may or may not be able to hear, but that doesn't mean that you should not talk to him or her. Go ahead and say all that you want or need to say to your loved one, assuming that your words will be heard.

Know what is written in the living will and durable power of attorney.

If your loved one has a current living will, that will specify the use of certain treatments. For example, the patient may decide that he or she doesn't want a feeding tube or IV fluids just to prolong life. Your loved one may also decide not to be resuscitated if his or her heart stops beating or to be put on a breathing machine. It's the patient's body, so he or she should be the one to make decisions about it.

A durable power of attorney will name someone to make health care decisions when your loved one is unable to do so, such as if he or she is in a coma. This includes what types of pain meds, how they are to be administered, what procedures may be performed, or anything else not specifically covered in the living will.

Be sure to discuss these with family members, so they will know what your loved one wants, whether specified in the advance directives or not. Choosing not to have aggressive medical treatment is different from refusing all medical care. The patient may still get pain meds, antibiotics, nutrition, and other treatments. However, at this stage, treatment is more for comfort than cure.

One thing to note: a living will may be revoked at any time, so if your loved one recovers from a coma, he or she can inactivate previous wishes. You and your loved one may want to have one in effect at all times, just in case something happens suddenly, such as a car accident that would render you incapable of making medical decisions.

Coma is peaceful.

Knowing he would slip into a coma and then into heaven was comforting to Bryan. He was concerned about pain, so we had worked out a system before he became comatose. He was receiving pain meds every four hours, but if he felt pain between doses, he would moan and I'd give him an extra pain pill. They were inserted into his rectum, so I would cut up a glycerin suppository and embed the pill into it. Then, the pill could be inserted quickly and painlessly, and would dissolve faster with the glycerin. Bryan would relax and lie quietly as the pain meds took effect.

When the end is near, breathing will become shallower and then stop completely. The breathing may stop one or more times before the end. This will give you a forewarning to gather around. Bryan's daughter Lisa was sitting with him when this happened, and she called me from the other room so we could both be with him when he passed. I will be forever grateful. It was very tranquil.

A coma can be a peaceful way to slip into eternity. It was for Bryan, and it may be for your loved one as well.

STEP 3—WHAT IS A DNR (DO NOT RESUSCITATE)?

A"Do Not Resuscitate" or DNR order may also be called a "Do Not Attempt Resuscitation" or DNAR.

Put the DNR in an envelope on the refrigerator door.

A DNR contains instructions that your loved one does not want anyone to try to revive him or her if the heart stops beating. In the hospital, a DNR sign will be posted in or just outside the room, so all personnel can see it. At home, the hospice nurse or doctor will put it in an envelope and hang it on the refrigerator door. Label the envelope "(State name) Directive" such as "Colorado Directive." This is where emergency personnel will look if called to your home.

Don't call 911 if there is a DNR.

There may be a moment of indecision when someone has called 911 and emergency medical technicians (EMTs) are at the door, expecting to resuscitate unless there is a DNR. We were told that if we called 911, Bryan would be put on a breathing machine, would be taken to the hospital and would not come home again. He didn't want that, so the DNR was in place to assure us that he would stay home and be comfortable.

As upsetting as it was to discuss DNR instructions for Bryan, the hospice doctor explained it very clearly. We understood what procedures could be done at home, in hospital, or by ambulance personnel, and the likelihood of their success. It helped us to make a more educated decision and feel better about it.

Make sure everyone knows about the DNR.

If your loved one has signed a DNR, be sure your family and all caregivers are aware, so that no unwanted procedures are performed by mistake. Give copies to the grown children and caregivers. If traveling with your loved one, check with your health care provider about state laws regarding having an original DNR or a duplicate on your person.

You don't need an attorney to craft a DNR. It only needs to be signed by the patient and one or more witnesses. Give a copy to the person named as your loved one's agent in his or her living will or durable power of attorney. Don't lock up the original in a safe deposit box, wall safe, or any other storage that only one or two people can open. It needs to be available on a moment's notice.

A friend told me about a medical alert bracelet for DNR that the patient can wear at all times. It will act only as an alert for medical personnel, but will not take the place of an official countersigned piece of paper. Even if your loved one wears the bracelet, be sure to have the paper accessible as well.

If at any time the patient changes his or her mind, be sure to let everyone know and destroy all copies of the DNR. Your loved one has control over what others do to his or her body, so be sure everyone involved knows what the patient wants every day. Take control when you can, and both you and your loved one will have more power in this journey.

STEP 4—WHAT DO WE DO
IF THE END COMES?

As the end of life nears, some people will gather the family around. If the patient has approved it, have family near to say goodbye and support one another. Some would rather not be around at the point of death; don't force them or make them feel guilty for not being there. You may regret it later.

Physical Changes

When death is near, your loved one may have physical changes:

- Less interest in food, sometimes not eating for days at the end.
- Trouble swallowing pills or medication. Ask your doctor if meds can be administered by IV or rectally instead. Cutting a glycerin suppository into 3-4 pieces and pushing a pill into one piece of glycerin makes it easier to insert rectally. It will then dissolve more rapidly than without the suppository.
- Extreme weakness. The patient needs help to get out of bed, move, or change position. Record any position changes in your notebook, such as when moving the patient from his or her back to the right side.
- Difficulty concentrating or confusion. Try to keep the atmosphere calm and quiet, maybe with soothing background music. You may want to limit visitors.
- Involuntary movements or jerking. Don't be alarmed, and don't talk about them in the same room. The patient may be aware and embarrassed by them.
- More drowsiness, especially with increased pain medication. Some patients will sleep for several days and may appear semi-comatose.

- Urine may be uncontrolled and dark in color. Use adult absorbent underwear and warn the patient when you're going to check or change him or her.
- Hands and feet may become blotchy or blue. Use extra blankets, not electric blankets, which can burn fragile skin.
- Changes in breathing patterns, such as noisy, moist breathing, called a "death rattle," which can be frightening if the patient is awake. Sitting up may help.

Make a List for Phone Calls

Make a list beforehand of all those you will want to call, including their telephone numbers. Your mind will be too fuzzy at the time to remember all of them. If possible, have someone with you to help with the calls and give support.

Ask loved ones ahead of time if they will want to see the body. Some will want to, while others will not want to be around the body. Most of our family did not want to see Bryan's body, as they had already said their goodbyes. Those who arrived at the house while his body was still there went to a separate room to wait.

When hospice is involved, they will know what to do and will give you a list of those to call at the time of death. Otherwise, talk with your doctor about what procedure to follow. Your first call should be to hospice or your doctor. They will send someone out to sign papers for the death certificate. Don't call 911, as there is nothing the emergency medical personnel can do.

Be prepared to spend a lot of time on the telephone. You may want to have at least one cell phone in addition to your landline, so you and your support person can make simultaneous calls. If possible, use two cell phones and keep your landline free for incoming calls.

Have your mortuary chosen and contacted ahead of time. One of your calls will be to the mortician, who will arrive soon, at a time you request. The mortician will bring a gurney (an ambulance bed) to carry your loved one. Two people will gently lift the body onto the gurney, cover with a blanket, and strap it on, just as if they were taking someone to the hospital. Some people prefer not to be in the room when the mortician lifts the body. Warn them ahead of time and let them do whatever they need.

When Bryan passed away, the mortician arrived before his assistant, so he gave me the option of waiting or helping. I chose to help Bryan one last time, and lifted his legs onto the gurney. Then I watched while the man gently wrapped a hand-stitched quilt around him and strapped him securely. It was a much more comforting ritual than I expected.

Death Certificates

The mortician will ask how many death certificates you want. Ask for at least ten; I got fourteen and so far have used eleven of them. Some entities will keep the original; others will make a copy and return the original to you.

You will need an original death certificate for:

- Social Security.
- Bank or credit union accounts.
- Car titles.
- Property held in joint tenancy.
- Stock transfer.
- Inherited property or stocks.
- Life insurance policies.
- The patient's children, stepchildren, or anyone mentioned in the will.
- Surviving parents, especially if the patient was mentioned in their wills.
- Nursing home account.
- Changing names on utilities or cell phone.
- Credit card companies.
- Medicare checks.
- Income tax if a refund is due.
- Any company the deceased had investments with.

Knowing what is coming and preparing for it can make the journey easier. Handling the death of a loved one is never easy, but being prepared can make this step more bearable.

STEP 5—PLANNING A FUNERAL OR MEMORIAL SERVICE

A funeral or memorial service is for the living, but it helps if the deceased had some say in it.

Make a List of Your Loved One's Favorites

Your loved one may have favorite:

- Songs that are special to him or her.
- Pictures or memories he or she wants shared.
- Clothing he or she wants to wear.
- People your loved one wants to sing at or conduct his or her service.

If your loved one's desires are only in his or her will, those directions may not be read until after the service. This would be devastating, knowing that a loved one's wishes weren't followed.

For the patient, it can be very comforting to know that these and other details are covered. Your loved one may realize what the future holds and want some input into it. Let your loved one have his or her say.

If you are notified that someone is going to pass away, take advantage of the opportunity. In fact, you might want to plan this when everyone is healthy, to find out what each person would like at his or her own service. Put it in writing, since you can't always rely on your memory when the time comes.

Celebrate Life

Instead of focusing on death, celebrate the life of your loved one. At Bryan's service, we had a video montage with photographs of his entire life, accompanied by songs that were special to him. We added captions to pictures that need explaining, such as names of others in the photo or describing the situation. Many friends learned things about Bryan they never knew and thanked me for the video.

We also had four people speak about memories of Bryan's life: his brother, his son and daughter, and me, his widow. His daughter Lisa and I wrote out what we wanted to say a few weeks ahead of time and read them to Bryan, which pleased him immensely. He then asked to see what we had written, so he could read for himself. He was delighted to know exactly how we felt and what we would be saying about him. It wasn't as hard as I thought to get up and talk at the service. I just focused on how I wanted everyone to remember him.

Share a Meal (and Hugs) Together

If possible, have a meal immediately after the service, so all the visitors will have the opportunity to stay and reminisce with you and with each other. Most churches will have a group of volunteers to provide food, setup, and cleanup, leaving you free to socialize and get much-needed hugs.

The meal doesn't need to be elaborate. After Bryan's service, our church provided ham sandwiches, salads, chips, and cookies. The leftovers went home with us to feed out-of-town guests. At my sister Barb's service, the food was potluck, with friends in her church donating a main dish, side dish, or dessert, spreading the cost around. Let your friends handle it for you.

If you want a graveside service, you may consider having it first, then returning to the church for a memorial. That way, you can have a meal afterward at the church without driving back and forth. You can limit the graveside service to immediate family and a few friends, and have everyone join you afterward.

Whatever you choose, spend as much time as you need with friends and loved ones. This may be the only chance you'll have today to visit and talk with them about your loved one, so take advantage of it.

STEP 6—BURIAL OR CREMATION?

Choosing between burial (also called interment) and cremation of your loved one's body is a personal choice. One is no better or worse than the other, unless there is a religious reason. The patient should have the final say.

Most people assume their body will be disposed of the way their family always has done it. However, that doesn't mean that you must follow suit. Look at all your options and make an educated decision.

Organ Donation

Be sure you know your loved one's wishes about organ donation. This may or may not be possible, especially if the patient is not hospitalized at the time of death, but be sure the family knows what the patient wants. A friend's eye tissue was harvested even though cancer had spread throughout his body. Allowing medical personnel to collect whatever can be used will help someone else live a fuller life.

Burial

When deciding between burial and cremation, cost is one consideration. A complete burial can cost thousands of dollars. Some include services like embalming, makeup and hair styling, a casket, a vault to hold the casket, transportation, opening and closing the grave, and a marker or headstone. Be aware that the mortician is in business and will try to up-sell you to a higher grade of casket, plot, or whatever. Take an uninvolved third party with you if possible to keep you from overspending in your moment of grief.

Your loved one's body will be transported to the mortuary or another location for treatment. After embalming, a specially trained beautician can add makeup and hairstyle to match a photograph provided by the family, making the deceased look as natural as possible. Makeup and hair styling are necessary only if there will be public viewing of the body.

The casket will need to be placed into a cement vault in the ground, to keep the casket from decaying. Some cemeteries also offer mausoleums, which are above-ground "drawers" in which the casket is placed. The face of the drawer contains the deceased's information, much like a headstone for a grave. Mausoleums are usually more expensive than an in-ground burial.

Some people want personal effects buried with them. If they are of no value, this may not be an issue. However, burying an expensive ring or other piece of jewelry can create problems in the family, especially when it was promised to someone. It is best to keep all valuables for sharing later.

Cremation

Cremation is a much cheaper alternative than burial. Your loved one's body will be transported to a location with a large oven. I saw a television documentary that described this as "light like the sun" surrounding your loved one. The body is reduced to ashes and bone fragments. These will weigh just a few pounds and can fit into a small box or urn.

With a minimal cremation, your loved one's remains will be returned to you in a plastic bag inside a small box, usually plastic. You can also purchase an urn for the ashes, which can be placed on a mantle or bookshelf. You can then feel that the loved one is still around. Decide what you'll do with the ashes, so you'll know what kind of container you want.

If your loved one wants his or her ashes spread somewhere, be sure to check local laws. Some states or municipalities have very strict rules about body disposal, and you don't want to break the law.

Combination Of Burial And Cremation

You can also do a combination of burial and cremation. A friend wanted her body cremated. However, she died suddenly and her husband felt the family needed a chance to say goodbye. Her body was prepared for viewing, and then cremated after the service. Unfortunately, he had to pay for embalming and purchase a casket, since these cannot be rented or reused.

Whatever you choose, be sure everyone in the family knows your decision. Bryan and I had decided on cremation years earlier, mainly due to the cost. We had told our children our decisions, but his mother wasn't aware until we were on our cancer journey. Since it was a last-minute surprise to her, it put me in the uncomfortable position of having to explain and justify it.

STEP 7—HOW DO I GRIEVE?

The best way to grieve is to let it out. Too many physical symptoms and ailments can be caused by internalizing one's feelings. You don't need sickness to add to everything else you're dealing with.

Coping With Grief

Here are some ways to cope with your grief:

- Cry. Tears have a way of cleansing and relieving internal pressure.
- Don't try to be strong all the time. Allow yourself to be human, to feel, and to let it out.
- Remember. Memories are our links to the past and we don't need to let them go. Moving on does not mean forgetting.
- Talk with a friend about your loved one. If your friend says it's time for you to quit talking, find another friend.
- Find comfort where you can. Listen to music or watch television shows or movies that you and your loved one enjoyed.
- Don't forget to eat. Don't overeat. If you let food become your comfort, it will only complicate things later.

I want to share one more time the five stages of grief, as stated by Elisabeth Kübler-Ross in her book *On Death and Dying*.[17]

Denial

This is when you can't believe what is happening. You may temporarily pretend that nothing has changed and that life will go on unaffected, one day at a time. You have probably gone past this stage since you're reading this book and are dealing with reality.

---

[17] http://grief.com/the-five-stages-of-grief/

Anger

This is where you scream and yell, "It's not fair!" "Why us?" "Who or what is to blame for this?" It's OK to feel the anger, but be careful that you don't inflict permanent damage to yourself or your relationships. See "Emotional Step 1—Dealing with anger" for tips on how to control this feeling.

Denial-Anger-Bargaining-Depression-Acceptance

Bargaining

This stage can come at any time in the journey. You start wondering if you or your loved one could have or should have done something different or if you can do something differently now. Maybe you could have altered the outcome or stopped the cancer from ever coming. This is the "What if..." game. It doesn't hurt to think of all the possibilities, but don't let them ruin your life.

Depression

This is the low point. Many of us have been there before, and it's not where we want to spend our lives. Talking with a loved one or a counselor or getting help from your doctor can reduce the extent of this stage.

Acceptance

You realize what's happened and prepare to do whatever is necessary. You tell yourself that everything will be OK and you can handle the outcome.

These steps don't always come in the same order, and you may need to repeat one or more, but they do present themselves at various points along the way. If you know they're coming, you can prepare for them and handle them better than if you're blindsided.

Hospice Offers Grief Counseling

Hospice has support and counseling for anyone grieving a loss. If your loved one was not in hospice, seek out a hospice in your area and enroll in their Newly Bereaved Support Class. This is for those who have lost a loved one within the previous three months. It was invaluable for me after Bryan's death, and it can help you get through this most difficult time. Hospice also offers ongoing support groups and counseling at minimal cost. Take advantage of any help offered.

Anniversaries, "monthiversaries," even "weekiversaries" will be especially hard, as will the time of death. After Bryan died, I wondered why I was miserable every Friday morning at 9:30, until I realized that was the time he died. The twenty-fourth of every month was hard for the same reason.

Allow yourself to grieve and feel your loss. If you know these times are coming, they won't blindside you and may be easier to deal with. When you find yourself especially weepy or depressed, ask yourself what this time, this day of the week, or this date meant with your loved one, and you will very likely find a connection.

Create New Memories

Create new memories for holidays or other special days. For the first Christmas after Bryan died, we had Santa Claus visit in person and bring gifts to all the grandchildren. It was actually a friend who portrays Santa and has a wonderful velvet suit. On the anniversary of Bryan's death, my mom spent the night before at my house and took me to breakfast. Then, my sister gave Colorado Avalanche hockey tickets to me, my son, and his wife for the game that night. I'm grateful for their thoughtfulness, and I was too busy to let the day get me down.

> **Don't risk dependence on "happy pills."**

If you're having a problem with depression, don't be afraid to ask your doctor for help. He may give you a 30-day prescription of a medication to help you on your worst days, but don't abuse it. Addiction isn't a fun thing to deal with, so don't let yourself go there. Taking a pill can impair your ability more than you think, and create more problems than you want to deal with, such as a DUI (Driving Under the Influence). Take medication when you'll be staying home.

I cut my "happy pills" in half, then in half again, and took only a fourth of a pill when I needed it. Then, I could take another fourth if needed and didn't run the risk of dependence. Using this method, two pills lasted four months.

If you feel you need more or stronger meds, consider counseling along with the pills. It's not a sign of weakness, but rather an indication that you realize what you need and are not afraid to get it.

Grief is a process.

Grief is a process, not an overnight action, and certainly not a place to stay indefinitely. Actively work on your grief and you can move through it. It won't happen in a day or even in a week. But you'll wake up one day and realize that you finally feel good again. Give it a chance.

STEP 8—LEARNING TO LIVE
A "NEW NORMAL" LIFE

Your life will never be the same. You have lost a loved one and must learn to live a "new normal" life, since your "old normal" life is gone. There is no right or wrong way to live and no exact timetable for getting past your grief. Grief must be worked through, not kept inside. It may take weeks, months, or even years. Give it as long as you need.

Try Not To Change Some Things

Some things in your life can stay the same, but others will change. Things that may help by not changing are:

- Staying in the same house and neighborhood.
- Shopping at the same grocery store.
- Parking your car in the same general area when you go shopping.
- Developing a daily routine.
- Going to bed and getting up at the same time every day, even on weekends.
- Maintaining relationships and finding time to get together with friends and family members.

Wait Two Years To Make Major Decisions

Major decisions, such as moving, remarrying, or changing jobs, should wait for at least a year, maybe two years. You are likely to make mistakes now, and you don't need them to be life-changing. If you're thinking of a major change, give it some time and discuss it with trusted friends and family members.

This timeline is not set in stone. Use your best judgment. Bryan and I met shortly after his wife died, and were married less than a year after her death. It was the best thing for both of us, and we had a wonderful marriage. A friend and her husband had been planning to move out-of-state to be near family when he was diagnosed. She decided to go ahead with their plan, moving just months after his death, and was happy she did. Another lonely friend remarried shortly after his wife died. Soon after that, he found himself divorced and alone.

Use your best judgment.

Use your best judgment when making emotional decisions. Talk with loved ones before making a major life change. Everyone is different, and what is right for one person may not be right for another.

Find ways of tricking your mind. A lamp in my living room is on a timer, set to turn off after I've gone to bed so I don't feel alone. At night, my extra bed pillows are on Bryan's side of the bed, so I can rest my hand where his chest used to be. Think of harmless ways to ease your transition. Then, when your new normal is in place, you can stop these little tricks.

You don't need to get rid of your loved one's clothes and possessions right away. There's no rush, so keep them around if you need them. You'll know when it's time to donate to charity. Take your time going through everything piece by piece, to be sure you don't get rid of something special you wanted to keep.

Your life will never be the same, but that doesn't mean it will always be bad. The "new normal" will be your new routine and will eventually feel OK.

STEP 9—DO I TALK ABOUT MY LOVED ONE OR JUST BE QUIET?

By all means, talk about your loved one. You have many good memories, and maybe some not-so-good ones, that need to be talked about, not kept inside.

Talk about your loved one.

Talking is the best way to work through your grief. Find a friend or family member whom you can trust with your deepest secrets, and ask the person if he or she will let you talk. Not everyone is a good listener, so choose wisely.

You may talk in person or over the phone if the person is some distance away. Schedule a time when you won't be interrupted. Find out if you can call the person at any hour, since you may need to talk in the middle of the night. You may find more than one person you trust, and be thankful for all of them. Talk as much and as often as necessary. If your friend tells you to stop talking, find another friend.

Write anything that comes to you.

If you prefer to write, get a journal or a notebook and let the words flow. This will be your private thoughts and feelings, so notate whatever you need to write. Don't worry about grammar or complete sentences. Just write. Keep the journal in a place where no one will find it unless you want them to read it. You can include photos of your loved one or memorable times with him or her, or draw a picture showing your emotions.

When Bryan and I married, he hadn't completed his grief work over his late wife, Beth. We would spend an evening each week discussing her over dinner and would sit for an hour or longer while Bryan reminisced. It helped both of us by letting him bare his soul about his feelings and allowing me to see his sensitivity. It drew us closer and cemented our relationship. It can do the same for you, if you find the right person to help you.

Write for yourself. Write for others.

You may want to write down your experiences for your personal reference. Or, you may want to help others by writing your story and sharing your memories, working through your own emotions in the process. That's what this book was for me—a chance to deal with the roller coaster of my feelings, knowing that this will help many people on their own journeys.

If you decide to create a book, a story, or a blog, learn how to write so others will want to read it. Just having a story doesn't guarantee that others will be interested. Attending writers' conferences and workshops helped make my book more readable, even though I was already writing.

Decide who your audience will be and write to them. Imagine them sitting in the same room and talk to them. Then find out how to get your story to those who may need it.

I'm convinced that God allows us to face terrible things so we can help others in similar situations. Turning your grief into something that can benefit others is the greatest testament to your loved one and the value of their life.

Please visit my website at *www.SteppingThroughCancer.com* for more help on your journey. Let me know how you're doing and if you decide to write your story. I'd love to read it. We're here to help each other.

STEP 10—KEEPING THE MEMORY ALIVE

Death does not mean we should forget a loved one. However, human memory has limitations, and we can help it out.

Pictures

Pictures, videos, and other images of our loved one can help us to remember. You don't need to surround yourself with pictures, but put them where you can see them when you need to. One wall in our living room has pictures of our grandchildren with a quote above them that says, "Count Your Blessings." After Bryan's death, I put an 8x10 photo of him in the middle, so he's surrounded by our grandkids, and he's one of the blessings I count every day.

Memories Wall

My website contains a Memories Wall with pictures and short biographies of loved ones who have fought cancer. Go to *SteppingThroughCancer.com*. Feel free to contact me at *bdhardy@msn.com* with a picture and a short bio of your loved one to add there.

Victories Wall

We also have a Victories Wall on my website for cancer survivors. Anyone can send me their picture with a 25-word story about their cancer journey, life before and since, or anything they would like the world to know about their fight. Go to *SteppingThroughCancer.com*.

Keep Recordings

Some people complain that they can't remember their loved one's voice. If you have a recording or voice mail of them, save it in multiple media, so you can listen whenever you need to. You could have it on tape and also recorded electronically so you can listen with a tape recorder or on your phone or computer.

Tangible Mementos

Honor your loved one with something tangible, such as planting a tree in his or her honor or donating to a cause he or she championed. Contact groups or organizations your loved one was passionate about and ask what they need. Then you can donate something other than money, like a piece of furniture or electronics. You could ask for a plaque near your donation inscribed with your loved one's name so others will remember him or her as well. If the entity would prefer a cash donation, ask if you can have a plaque or sign somewhere acknowledging your loved one's gift.

You may want to preserve your loved one's room or a part of the house he or she used just as he or she left it. As long as you don't need the space for something else, there's no problem. Many parents have kept a child's room exactly as it was for months or years. A wife may keep the workbench in the garage the way her husband used it last. In fact, I can't bring myself yet to let our sons and son-in-law take some of Bryan's tools. Maybe someday I will, but not just yet.

Remember, But Don't Live in Your Memories

Remember your loved one, but don't let the memory control your present and your future. You're still alive, and you have the chance to make the most of your life in honor of your loved one. Take advantage of opportunity before you, thanking your loved one for the experience of having him or her in your life. We only have one chance to live, and today is your chance.

APPENDICES

HOW TO USE THE APPENDICES

The following appendices include some ideas for patients, some for care-givers, and some for family and friends. I provided these to help deal with the cancer, with the situation, and with each other. There are separate lists for each group. The last two were combined since the line between family and friends can become blurred. We have so many friends that are more like family, and you probably do as well.

Feel free to make copies of any appendix you need and give it to someone who needs the ideas. Those who don't have this book may not know how to act, what to say, or how to help. You can give them ideas of how to help you by telling them what you need.

Appendix D lists additional resources if you choose to do some research on your own. I highly recommend my editor Hope's website, *www.SeeHope. com*, as a resource to find hope (no pun intended) and peace. (Her name is C. Hope, hence *SeeHope*.)

Many who have completed their own cancer journeys have wanted to tell their stories. Please do! There are over a million Americans with cancer[18], and they, along with their caregivers, can use all the encouragement they can find. Appendix E will give you some thoughts on writing effectively so others will read it.

Let me know how you're doing. Go to my website at *www. SteppingThroughCancer.com* to contact me. Many others also want to hear your success stories. We're here to help each other.

God bless you on your journey.

---

[18] *http://www.cancer.org/acs/groups/cid/documents/webcontent/002813-pdf.pdf*

APPENDIX A—HINTS FOR PATIENTS

1. Learn all you can about your cancer. Knowledge is power, so arm yourself for the fight.

2. Confide in a trusted friend or loved one, not necessarily your caregiver.

3. Get a loose-leaf notebook to hold all your bills, brochures, notes from every appointment, and questions to ask your doctor.

4. Take someone with you to appointments to write down all that is said.

5. Eat what you can when you can to keep up your strength.

6. If you are nauseated or getting chemotherapy, don't eat your favorite foods. Save them for when your stomach won't reject them.

7. Sleep when you can.

8. Laugh as much as possible. Watch funny movies or sitcoms on television.

9. Take advantage of a chance to get out for some fresh air.

10. Accept only visitors you want. You don't need to see everyone.

11. Follow all your oncologist's instructions and keep every appointment.

12. Get in touch with your spirituality. Read your Bible, pray, or meditate.

13. Never give up! You're worth fighting for, so keep fighting.

14. Write your feelings in a journal. Don't keep everything inside.

15. Ask for help. It shows wisdom, not weakness.

16. Advance health directives are a form of control, not a sign of surrender.

APPENDIX B—HINTS FOR CAREGIVERS

1. "If you find it in your heart to care for somebody else, you will have succeeded." Maya Angelou[19]

2. Get help. Don't try to do it all by yourself. Accept help if offered.

3. Prepare a loose-leaf notebook with tabs for notes, bills, meds (info from the pharmacist), medical info (from the web), questions to ask the doctor, and encouragement from friends or family.

4. Make a list of things friends can do and tell them when they ask.

5. Tell friends and family what is happening.

6. Confide in a trusted friend or loved one.

7. Find ways to laugh. Watch comedy movies or sitcoms on television.

8. Encourage the patient to eat, but don't force it.

9. Have the patient's favorite snacks within reach.

10. Get enough rest. Learn to nap if you can't sleep all night.

11. Find "me time" when possible. Ask a friend to stay with the patient while you shop, drive around, or just sit in your car.

12. Exercise produces energy. Try to work out a few minutes each day.

---

[19] http://brainyquotes.com/quotes/authors/m/maya_angelou_2.html

13. Spend time every day reading your Bible, praying, or meditating.

14. Keep the gas tank full and a tote bag by the door with a sweater, water bottle, paper and pen, cash, and cell phone cord for a run to the ER.

15. Regulate visitors. You don't need to let everyone come, especially if it may upset the patient.

16. Find a way to safely express your anger, depression, grief, or other emotions.

17. Filter bad news to the patient with care. Let others know if you have not told your loved one bad news such as Uncle Joe's passing, so they don't accidentally spill the beans.

18. Advance health directives are a form of control, not a sign of surrender for the patient. Encourage the patient to have his or her directives in place, and you do the same.

APPENDIX C—HINTS FOR FAMILY AND FRIENDS

1. Keep in contact. Don't cut off communication.

2. Send written encouragement, such as cards, letters, and e-mails. A phone call is nice, but something written can be read whenever support is needed.

3. Offer specific help, such as, "I'd like to bring dinner. What day would be best?" or, "I feel like cleaning. May I come and vacuum for you?" If you just say, "Let me know what I can do," the patient and caregiver won't know what you're willing to do and won't ask.

4. Find out what the patient can eat, and bring it.

5. Provide food that can be frozen and reheated, so it won't spoil before it can be eaten. Give reheating instructions.

6. Ask what the caregiver and patient need and want.

7. Call before visiting. Don't just drop in unannounced.

8. If you really mean that your loved one can call you any time, day or night, tell him or her so and offer your cell phone number.

9. Understand that you may show up at an inconvenient or awkward time and may be asked to leave, even if you called first. Don't take it personally.

10. Laugh with the patient and caregiver. Take a funny movie or a game and spend time.

11. Don't tell the patient and caregiver how strong they are, making them feel they can't show emotion around you.

12. Let the patient and caregiver talk. Let them cry. Learn to listen.

13. Allow the patient, caregiver, or other loved one to grieve in your presence.

14. Don't spread what you hear.

15. If you have a close relationship with the patient, offer to sit with him or her while the caregiver goes shopping or just gets away for some much-needed "me time."

APPENDIX D—ADDITIONAL RESOURCES

Here are some websites that I've found to be reliable:

- American Cancer Society *www.cancer.org*
- National Cancer Institute *www.cancer.gov*
- National Center for Complementary and Alternative Medicine *www.nccam.nih.gov*

And some that are not specifically for cancer:

- Answers.com *www.answers.com*
- MedicineNet.com *www.medicinenet.com*
- National Institutes of Health *www.nih.gov* (this has 27 health entities)
- National Library of Medicine *www.nlm.nih.gov*
- WebMD *www.webmd.com*

Peace and hope for the future:

- Hope Flinchbaugh's website *www.seehope.com*
- My website *www.SteppingThroughCancer.com.*

APPENDIX E—WRITING YOUR STORY

You may want to help others by writing your story and sharing your memories, working through your own emotions in the process. That's what this book was for me—a chance to deal with my roller coaster of feelings, knowing that this will help many people on their journeys. Write your story no matter what the ending. People need to know how you got where you are, especially if you found joy in spite of the cancer.

If you decide to create a book, a story, or a blog, please learn how to write so others will want to read it. Just having a story doesn't guarantee that others will be interested. I attended writers' conferences and workshops, even though I was already writing, to hone my abilities and make my books more readable.

Picture your audience and write to them. You may want to imagine someone in particular sitting next to you and just write to them. That's what I did—I pictured a friend helping her husband through cancer treatments and talked to her. That makes it much more personal and easier to write. Then, find out how to get your story to those who may need it.

I'm convinced that God allows us to face terrible things so we can help others in similar situations. Turning your success or grief into something that can benefit others is the greatest way to honor or remember your loved one and give value to his or her life.

The previous appendices will give you some specific hints for caregivers, patients, family members, and friends, as well as other resources. Most people do not know intuitively how to handle cancer when it affects them personally. These suggestions could take out some of the speed bumps and potholes in your journey and make life a little easier.

Please visit my website at *www.SteppingThroughCancer.com* for more help on your journey. Let me know how you're doing and if you decide to write your story. I'd love to read it. We're here to help each other. I hope this book has helped you, and you in turn can help others.

God bless you on your journey.

NOTE FROM THE AUTHOR

Stepping through cancer isn't easy. I'd love to hear about you or your loved one and share in your journey as you've allowed me to share mine. If you have questions or just need to talk, you can find me at *www. SteppingThroughCancer.com*. This is a road best traveled with friends.

IF YOU'RE A FAN OF THIS BOOK, PLEASE TELL OTHERS...

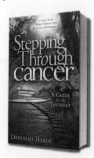

- Write about *Stepping Through Cancer* on your blog, Twitter, MySpace, and Facebook page.
- Suggest *Stepping Through Cancer* to friends.
- When you're in a bookstore, ask if they carry the book. The book is available through all major distributors, so any bookstore that does not have *Stepping Through Cancer* in stock can easily order it.
- Write a positive review of *Stepping Through Cancer* on *www.amazon.com*.
- Send my publisher, HigherLife Publishing, suggestions on websites, conferences, and events you know of where this book could be offered at *media@ahigherlife.com*.
- Purchase additional copies to give away as gifts.

CONNECT WITH ME...

To learn more, visit my website at *www.SteppingThroughCancer.com* or email me at debbie@steppingthroughcancer.com.

You may also contact my publisher directly:

HigherLife Publishing
400 Fontana Circle
Building 1 – Suite 105
Oviedo, Florida 32765
Phone: (407) 563-4806
E-mail: *media@ahigherlife.com*

INDEX

Item / Step   Page

Item / Step	Page

Item / Step Page

Item / Step	Page